MUSIC AND MENTAL HEALTH
Let's Talk About Emo

MUSIC AND MENTAL HEALTH
Let's Talk About Emo

Written By:
Brey Dawson
Jessica Jutras
Austin Mardon
Robert Mcweeny
Zach Schauer
Riley Witiw

Cover Design By:
Josh Harnack

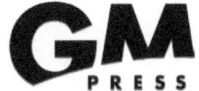

Copyright © 2020 by Austin Mardon

All rights reserved. This book or any portion thereof may not be reproduced or used in any manner whatsoever without the express written permission of the publisher except for the use of brief quotations in a book review or scholarly journal.

First Printing: 2020

Typeset and Cover Design by Josh Harnack

ISBN: 978-1-77369-179-4

Golden Meteorite Press
103 11919 82 St NW
Edmonton, AB T5B 2W3
www.goldenmeteoritepress.com

Table of Contents

Introduction 11
Part One: Radio Silence… Mostly 17
    Classical's Falling Empire 18
    The Jams of North America 23
        Blues 23
        Country 25
        Jazz 27
    Folk, Rock, and Things You Don't Discuss at the Dinner Table 30
    Soda and All That Other Fizz 37
Part Two: Cheer Up, Emo Kid 45
    First Wave: Softboiled Hardcore Toughguys 46
    Second Wave: We Like Choruses Now 52
    Third Wave: The Coolest Losers in the World 56
    Media's Response (Not Huge Fans) 65
    … Moral Panic (Pt. II) 76
Part Three: Out of the Moshpit, Into the Clinic, then Back to the Moshpit ... 83
    Did Music Save My Life? 84
    Fourth Wave: Defending Pop-Punk: Sliding Into the 2010s on a Pizza Skateboard 90
    Fifth Wave: Emo but with 808s This Time 103
Part Four: The After Effects of the Scene 109
    Increasing Rapport for Group Support 110
    Everyone is Emo Now 123
    The Crown Jewel: Musical Therapy 133
        Music therapy: our scientific understandings 134
        Music Therapy and Mental Health 137
Conclusion 139

e·mo
/ˈēmō/

Noun: emo; noun: emo-core; noun: emocore

A style of rock music resembling punk but having more complex arrangements and lyrics that deal with more emotional subjects.

- an admirer of emo music or a member of the subculture associated with it.

plural noun: emos

- "I'm not one of those emos who are always crying—I just want to make that clear"

Derived from "emotional hardcore" in the 90s.

Adjective: emo

denoting or relating to emo and its associated subculture.

- "an emo band"

See Also:

Emo is a broad, hard to pin-down type of word. It is sometimes synonymous with punk-rock music, or pop-punk music. Sometimes it is used in a slanderous and derogatory way. It defines a subculture and a social movement. Basically: every year, every generation, every individual has their own definition of Emo.

> "I've never recognized 'emo' as a genre of music. I always thought it was the most [stupid] term ever. I know there is this generic commonplace that every band that gets labeled with that term hates it. They feel scandalized by it. But honestly, I just thought that all the bands I played in were punk rock bands. The reason I think it's so stupid is that—what, like the Bad Brains weren't emotional? What—they were robots or something? It just doesn't make any sense to me."
> - *Guy Picciotto, lead singer of Rites of Spring*

> "I get what people are saying with the eyeliner and the girl pants and this and that. Hopefully, [emo] is more than just a T-shirt slogan... For a long time, we talked about playing in front of a giant banner that said 'EMO.' If you're emo, you might as well be in on the joke."
> - *Pete Wentz, bassist of Fall Out Boy*

> "Emo is a pile of shit."
> - *Gerard Way, lead singer of My Chemical Romance*

> "To some, the sound of hardcore music with impassioned lyrics is the end-all and be-all of emo. This view mistakes musical moment for genre. Emo is the soundtrack to youth, and as times change, so does the music that resonates with young people. The history of emo is one of reinvention and bigger and bigger stages—of shifting musical styles and baggage across generations."
> - *Andy Greenwald, in 'Nothing Feels Good: Punk Rock, Teenagers, and emo.'*

"To me and my friends, emo was always synonymous with hardcore. I think it's relative to where you grew up, what these words—punk, hardcore, emo—mean. If you grew up in Southern California you're going to have a much different definition of hardcore than if you grew up on Long Island. So, to us, emo and hardcore meant the same thing, really. Bands like Julia, Indian Summer, and Current. They were emo."
- Jim Adkins, lead singer of Jimmy Eat World

"Emo is inherently inclusive... Better together than alone."
- Andy Greenwald, in 'Nothing Feels Good: Punk Rock, Teenagers, and emo.'

INTRODUCTION

The past decade has seen the emergence of mental health as one of the most prominent topics in media, whether that discourse occurs in news outlets announcing new medications, university students flooding psychology departments with enrollments, or hashtags on all social media platforms promoting mental health awareness of all types. Crisis hotline numbers are a Google search away, along with resources, research, information, statistics, advice, and support. Before the internet, most of this dissemination would be impossible.

Yet we cannot credit the internet with the spread of mental health conversation since the web only contains the topics that people want to talk about. Any other talking point could occupy the blogs and website domains that are instead filled with mental health discussion. So, why is it today that mental health is so widely discussed, and so surprisingly accepted, especially by younger audiences?

We want to examine one contributing factor to this movement, and though it may seem like an unlikely contender to anyone ignorant of it, we think that this contributing factor is emo music. We will leave the question, "what is emo music?" until the second part of this book because it is a loaded question that requires context to answer. Besides, we need to establish, as we attempt in part one, that mental health was not receiving attention in other mainstream forms of music before we can claim that emo music was in any way unique.

Another question a reader might ask is: "why music?" In other words, even if it's true that mental health was not at the forefront of mainstream music until emo, why would music contribute to contemporary popularity of mental health conversations?

The short answer is: because almost everyone listens to music. Countless first-hand accounts from strangers on the street will confirm that music largely influences our lives. Public transit is stuffed with commuters listening to their favorite tunes before a long day at work or school; music plays in the background at almost every public place; and radio, streaming, and concerts are some of the largest forms of entertainment. At the gym, we listen to music. While we walk, we listen to music. When we invite friends over, we listen to music. In the car, we listen to music. You get the point. It doesn't take an academic statistical analysis of how people spend their leisure time to intuitively know that music is everywhere in modern society.

Further, musicians are celebrities, accumulating money-spending fan bases in the blink of an eye. Musicians are also often role models, idols, and exemplars for people of all ages. Everywhere we go, we find people wearing t-shirts, hoodies, hats, and other forms of merchandise that rep their favorite musicians. These people often defend their tastes in music, and are often willing to go as far as to claim that their favourite artists simply are the best. There is always some guy willing to deductively prove that Metallica is, as a stable, objective matter of fact, the best band ever. Period.

So, we decided that investigating the prevalence of mental health related music alongside the rise of mainstream mental health awareness was not a bad start to understanding why we love talking about our minds so much today.

The following manuscript is an introductory investigation into the relation of modern music (the 1900s and beyond) to mental health. We hope to elucidate how artists became more comfortable talking about mental health as time progressed into the 21st century. If the hunch we are examining is correct, then the rise of mental health in mainstream popular music and media is largely attributable to the concurrent rise of emo music as a best-selling and mainstream subculture.

Now, because our scope is unfathomably broad, we do not come close to exhausting any of the history, music, or media that we examine throughout this book. Further, we don't intend to follow a strict methodology, such as the scientific method or a standard literature review. Instead, we use content analysis, interviews, anecdotes, and general observations to try and string together the preliminary research needed to determine emo's role in sparking contemporary mental health discussions.

There are also a few other major limitations to this text we must bring forth:

The first limitation is that we will move through historical musical movements in the first part of this book. Since emo music takes its roots in traditional rock music, our historical analysis only tracks the lineage of rock and rock-related movements. There are three consequences of this focus. One, our historical traces leave entire movements and genres of music out the equation because they are too tangential or too much to fit in this book. Two, we necessarily reduce all of the genres of music to representative examples. In other words, we allow a few people to stand in for their whole movement or genre. There will always be exceptions to any established rule, so we wish to use more well-known, influential artists that more readers and researchers are familiar with rather than obscure and under documented artists. Finally, there are a few genres that we mention but do not give nearly enough attention, specifically blues and hip-hop. These two genres are too large to examine without going off topic, and they are so tightly knit within a lineage of history that mainstream rock and roll diverts from. We will just take it as an assumption that hip-hop had a profound influence on and a complex relationship with emo music.

The second limitation is our analysis and interpretation of song lyrics throughout this investigation. We recognize that the interpretation of any work of art is arduous and rigorous and that many, if not all, of the works we examine deserve more justice than we give them in this text. We also know that our interpretations are not the final and ultimate reading of the songs. There are many types of lyrical and musical analysis performed by many different brilliant minds and we do not dare to pretend to contend with them. We offer quicker, nitty-gritty style analysis that only discuss songs insofar as they relate to the subjects at hand.

Now a reader might be thinking: "So wait, let me get this straight. You want to study how mental health historically progresses in music, yet you've done bad history and bad musical analysis... why exactly should I read this book?"

Well, our method isn't bad — it just doesn't give a full story. The reason we have to conduct our research under such limitations is that there is no in-depth research on most of the topics we are examining — especially our main focus, emo music. Our attempts will only lay the groundwork for further inquiry into the individual artists, songs, eras, genres, and events that we pursue. Hopefully, we inspire some others to start reflecting on our questions with us.

We examine the book in four parts, which allows readers to consult specific historical moments and topics, while also maintaining a narrative-like structure for anyone who wishes to read front to back. The first part examines popular musical movements before emo. The second part examines the first three waves of emo, which are now in the past, and takes a look at how mainstream media responded to it. The third part investigates how emo responded to media responding to emo. The fourth part takes a look at the impact emo has had in our contemporary culture to promote mental health.

Finally, we want this read to be enjoyable and thought-provoking, so we (try to) keep a sense of humour throughout the book. It is typical of emo to be self-reflexive and ironic, so, in the spirit of emo, we follow in that vein of ironic humour. We also want our readers to understand the references we make and become familiar with our ideas. So, we provide suggested listenings at the start of each chapter to give context and encourage the reader to engage and think about emo.

Let's tune in, chill out, and get sad. It's gonna be a fun ride.

PART ONE: RADIO SILENCE... MOSTLY

Classical's Falling Empire

Recommended Listens:

1. Ode to Aphrodite (Original Composition For Replica Lyre in the Ancient Greek Hypodorian Mode) - Michael Levy
2. Kitharis - Petros Tabouris Ensemble, Petros Tabouris
3. The Rite of Spring: Part Two: The Sacrifice: Glorification of the Chosen One - Igor Stravinsky, Teodor Currnetzis, Musica Aeterna
4. Symphony No. 40 in G minor, K. 550: I. Molto allegro - Wolfgang Amadeus Mozart, Riccardo Minasi, Ensemble Resonanz
5. A Canadian Boat Song - Jim Krause

Western classical music is hard to define, especially considering the fact that the term refers to a long string of historical eras, genres, musical instruments, and political and artistic movements. Briefly put, classical music is the music rooted in major Western cultural traditions. The Western cultural traditions are just as difficult to precisely define but can be expressed as the practices, worldviews, and cultures of different time periods within the Western world. Finally, the Western world, once again, is hard to define. So, we will consider the Western world to be European and North American world, although our musical focus will remain primarily on America, Canada, and the United Kingdom because these cultures, and especially their musical traditions, are tightly linked and mutually influence each other to a large degree. We cannot do justice to the vast amounts of research in the field of Western music, nevermind the vast amounts of diversity and research on other worldly traditions. Therefore, we will relegate ourselves to a small little corner, painting broader brush strokes to stay focused on our topic — how music talks about mental health.

A brief (and incomplete) timeline of Western classical music would run as follows: Ancient Music falls anywhere before 500 A.D. and includes Ancient Greek, Roman, and Egyptian music — the scales and time signatures of which became the foundation of Western music. The Early Music period came next, encompassing the Medieval period of 500 to 1420 A.D., which focused on liturgical music, and the Renaissance of 1400 to 1600, which saw the rise of secular vocal and instrumental music. Finally, the common-practice period, which is united more by technical features than historical dates, arose after the Renaissance. Common-practice music is a goal oriented form, which uses melodies, rhythms, and counterpoint to achieve their desired goal (usually the goal is an idea or representation of something).

At the beginning of the 20th century, the Western world was expanding in one sense and getting smaller in another. It was expanding, on the one hand, due the near-complete colonization of North America. On the other hand, the more westerners explored, travelled, searched, and conquered, the less there was for them to discover.

Music has always been connected to any society's root culture and constitutes one of the most accessible, celebrated, and primordial forms of cultural expression. As the west expanded its physical geography, they wished to pass on their heritage and traditions to the new generations of the new world. Therefore, much of the musical tradition handed down in North America stemmed from the history of classical music that originated in and thrived in Europe, which stemmed from the traditional music of Greek tradition.

Yet there was a problem. The European empires and monarchies were dissolving, or at least losing their power and lustre, and members of the new societies wanted to distinguish themselves from the European ancestors. The European world could not control the North American world unfolding on the other side of the ocean.

As a consequence of this separation between the old western world and the new one, music began to become increasingly individualized by each nation, as the rise of national anthems and folk-based classical exploded onto the musical scene in the early 1900s. Here began a rebellion against classical music.

The rebellion against classical meant pushing back against the standards, values, forms, and theories of classical forms of music. Further, this rebellion involved an explosion of new genres and schools of music, which all tried, in one way or another, to separate themselves from the traditional elements of classical. Part of this separation was to engage in new subject matter, rather than the political, philosophical, and religious subjects that often dominated historically.

Much of the canonical classical music of the 20th century was not composed by North Americans and most of the canonical classical music responded to the waves of music that came before it. Also, many of the new nations had a never-before wielded creative power over their culture and the new traditions it would form. So, national anthems were the first stepping stones new nations and colonies used to create their unique cultures from scratch.

Now, there were also other forms of music arising in the new west — specifically in America. However, Canada did see a few big cultural songs written in its early years, though most of the records and transcriptions have not survived. Additionally, much of the Canadian folk music was written by non-Canadians and even people who were not immigrating, such as the famous "A Canadian Boat Song" written by the Irishman Thomas Moore in 1804.

Indeed, the uprising of music in the newly colonized west was far more impactful in the United States than in Canada. Americans had the regular ammunition of anthems and folk tunes and quickly saw the Spiritual, a form of call-and-response worship songs written and sung by the influx of slaves forced to work in America.

Now, given this incredibly brief and reductive history of music, we can begin to see that the modern idea of mental health simply was not a topic of conversation within the realms of music in the mainstream and high society. There were plenty of valid, intriguing, and important aesthetic movements throughout the ages, but none were focused directly on talking about mental health as we conceive it today.

Nonetheless, there were plenty of seeds that the classical western music planted, which would eventually blossom into a many-branched tree of different styles and genres, which would bear the fruit of many musicians to come.

The first of these seeds stretch far back in time to ancient Greece in the form of a stringed instrument in the yoke-lute family — the lyre. The lyre was the ancient Greek instrument used to accompany musical poetry that attempts to express emotions and feelings (opposed to religious praise), often in the first person. This emotional poetry accompanying the lyre became known as lyric poetry, which is where we derive the term "lyric" for the sung, spoken, screamed, or otherwise uttered words that accompany music.

Furthermore, the kithara (or in Latin, Cithara) was a species of lute with seven strings made for professional musicians. The kithara, through many variations over two thousand years, eventually became, and was renamed in English, the guitar. Combined with the idea of lyric poetry in which people sing in the first person about their feelings, the kithara player is the ancient Greek rendition of the singer-songwriters that we know today. The only difference is that the Greek lyrist was writing cool love songs and showing their soft sides before it was trendy.

The tradition of lyric poetry set to music that depicts inner feelings and emotions was the first step to the modern conversations about mental health that appear in music. This tradition carried on through the ages, and we can find many variations of the lute and lyric poetry from musicians and writers throughout the ages and the world: the Greek poet, Sappho; the medieval Franscesco Petrarch; Robert Ferrick in the Early Modern period; and the Romantic poets Percy Shelley and John Keats, to barely mention a few.

Another seed contributed by the prehistoric and ancient musicians, which may seem trivial to us today, is the modes and scales of musical theory they used. The theory of the ancients eventually developed into the theory of Western music that is still found in almost every contemporary song. Even modern music that doesn't use ancient theory is usually influenced by it because the modern avant-garde or futurist musician attempting to invent new modes and rhythms is responding to and rebelling against the ancient forms.

Further, even the ancients, and musicians before and after them, knew the effects that different modes of music can cause. In fact, in Plato's Republic, Socrates and his interlocutors discuss the best modes of music, and conclude that the lyre and the cithara are the best instruments because they are typically played in the modes suitable to promote courage and moderation. This example shows that even ancients were discussing the variety of emotions that music can reflect. Eventually, people began using music to encapsulate their feelings and emotions regarding mental health — and even try to give an impression on the experience of mental illness, though these uses of music were not on the horizon at this point in time. However, the ship had begun to sail with the invention of lyric poetry and the instruments that accompanied it.

The Jams of North America

Blues

Recommended Listens:

1. Stumble - Freddie King
2. You Don't Love Me - Little Walter, Bo Diddley, Muddy Waters
3. We The People - Guitar Shorty
4. Why I Sing The Blues - B.B King
5. Things I Forgot To Do - The Fabulous Thunderbirds

Blues music appeared in the late 1800s to the early 1900s, arising specifically around the time of the American Civil War. Founded on the field music and chants of West African slaves brought to America, blues began as an African-American genre expressing depressive moods experienced by the unbelievably traumatic experiences of slavery.

The experience of slavery cannot be underestimated as an influence on the development of the genre. Many of the old musical traditions of slaves fell apart during or worse, were banned. For example, American slave owners banned the use of drums, an important aspect of many African musical traditions, and forced slaves to convert to Christianity, further limiting slave self-expression by restricting musical subject matter.

Slaves were also refused education by governments, plantation owners, and the institutions, so other modes of artistic expression, such as painting and poetry, were often inaccessible. Regardless of English literacy and a lack of formal education, slaves needed an artistic outlet, and began inventing their own secular musical genre — the blues.

Generally, one can expect to find two broad subtypes of the blues. "Deep Blues," often considered the most elemental form of the blues, doesn't often see above-ground. Deep blues aren't as slow and mournful as one might expect. The subgenre is intense; spiteful, angry, pathos, and upbeat. Examples of deep blues include Little Walter's juke-joint harp blasts, Otis Rush's discography, and politically charged compositions from Guitar Shorty's, "We the People." Sure, you can dance to the beat, but the lyrics are often considered miserable.

The other branch of the blues is really just "rhythm and blues." It's what you hear from **B.B King**, the Fabulous Thunderbirds, and Freddie King. It's about every man's life, and frankly, it's relatable. It's simple, innocuous, and isn't particularly heavy emotionally or musically.

These sub-genres of blues are rooted in religious music, and this characteristic is demonstrable in its ability to make people "zone out" by listening to Blues' repetitive, catchy hooks, in much the way they might while listening to an extended spiritual mantra.

Generations of slaves relying on the blues to supplant woes and strife has been rigorously studied in modern times. We are now beginning to understand the scientific basis for the blues as an antidote to mental health conditions such as depression and anxiety. 8 and 12-bar blues patterns invoke changes of brain chemistry that are shown to reduce anxiety, and when utilized therapeutically, may help cure depression. These passages are digestible enough for our brain to actively interpret them, while being simple enough to not require pain-staking analysis.

That being said, there is also evidence to suggest that overtly depressing lyrical content may stifle blues music's efficacy as a therapeutic tool. Alas, the blues proves to be a relational swiss-army-knife that helps people contend with stark, crushing circumstances.

Country

Recommended Listens:

1. I think I'm Gonna Kill Myself - Buddy Knox
2. Good day - Brett Eldredge
3. Bridges - Mickey Guyton
4. Secondhand Smoke - Kelsea Ballerini
5. What Are You Gonna Tell Her? - Mickey Guyton
6. Humble and Kind - Tim McGraw
7. Better Days - Faith Hill
8. Hurt - Johnny Cash
9. If I Die Young - The Band Perry

The early 1900s saw the formation of country music, a uniquely American style of music that originated from Western European folk songs, and collided with blues and gospel influence around World War II. The lyrics of the time, decidedly melancholic and shrouded in nostalgia, spanned topics such as poverty, orphans, failing relationships, and loneliness. The lyrics were typically conveyed through the lens of a narrative, earning country music a reputation as the epitome of musical story-telling.

In more recent times, the sound and content of country music has evolved while still reflecting its grass roots. Largely, the music is written about love and relationships, but, since the 1960s, has shifted away from failing relationships to celebrating love. Similarly, another prominent topic in country music, regret and loss, has faltered in recent times in favour of songs that promote folk wisdom and traditional lifestyles.

However, when it comes to mental health, the amount of discourse within country music is minimal. For those versed in country music culture, this lack of discussion comes as no surprise. The genre is infamous for it's silence on hard-pressing issues, and artists who break that convention (ala the Dixie Chicks and their callout of George W. Bush in 2003) often alienate their fan bases. Consequently, many country artists are fearful to say anything their audience would construe as polarizing.

The occasional instances when mental health comes up are often mired by a tongue-in-cheek shroud — especially earlier on in the development of country music. One such example is the song, "I Think I'm Gonna Kill Myself," written by Buddy Knox in 1958, wherein the titular line is sang in a jaunty, upbeat melody that invites the listener to laugh away the gravitas of the notion. "Well I bow my head / 'Cause in the mornin' I'm a-gonna be dead / Yes, I think I'm gonna kill myself / I think I'm gonna kill myself," Knox gleefully sings. Similarly, Stringbean's 1967 track, "Suicide Blues," features a protagonist who facetiously explores several methods of suicide and fantasizes about his ex-lover's reaction upon learning that her departure was the direct cause. While these songs may seem crass and potentially unhelpful, it is possible these artists were attempting to explore taboo topics without making a statement that would come across as obscene to the country audencies of the mid 20th century. Regardless, they helped set a precedent that has only been notably broken in recent times in country music.

During the 2010s and its increasing general awareness of mental health, country music followed suit. One popular artist, Brett Eldredge, has written songs that engage in open, honest discussions of the experience of mental illness, in addition to promoting mental health events and initiatives. Other country artists like Kelsea Ballerini and Mickey Guyton have done the same. Still, these artists are relatively new and haven't quite achieved superstardom within their musical niche. There are exceptions to this rule: Tim McGraw with his songs, "Live Like You Were Dying," and "Humble and Kind;" also Faith Hill with songs like "Better Days."

Unfortunately, the indifferent disposition of country music towards mental health could be having a negative effect on it's listeners. One study found a statistically significant correlation between suicide rates and the prevalence of radio airtime devoted to country music opposed to other kinds of music in 49 large metropolitan areas. Of course, correlation is not necessarily causation, but this study does add to an increasing body of evidence which underscore the need for better mental health dialogue within country.

Jazz

Recommended Listens:

1. In A Sentimental Mood - Duke Ellington,
2. Summertime - Charlie Parker
3. Blue in Green - Miles Davis

To narrowly define jazz is an impossibility. The genre is staggeringly large and encompasses a history of over 100 years, beginning somewhere during the early 20th century. Between 1920 and 1940, jazz exploded in popularity alongside names such as Duke Ellington, Charlie Parker, and Miles Davis. Jazz is unique in that a performer has the freedom to respond to their environment through their style, tone, and ideas, and structure due to the genre's emphasis on improvisation. Consequently, a great deal of the music is non-lyrical, telling stories using nothing more than a sonic soundscape and a title to contextualize a song's narrative or message.

It may be that jazz and its improvisational qualities may be the direct result of mental illness, according to Dr. Sean Spence, a faculty member of the department of psychiatry at the University of Sheffield. Dr. Spence says that ragtime player Charles "Buddy" Bolden's schizophrenia impeded him from playing the correct notes in his performances. Therefore, Bolden would improvise his own parts, starting the phenomenon of jazz entirely by accident. These beginnings would seem to foreshadow many of the mental health struggles that jazz musicians would go on to face and write about in their music.

The lyrical topics of jazz music are wildly eclectic: love, everyday triumphs, sex, money, cooking, drinking, infedlity, and abuse have all found their way into jazz. Mental health, particularly addiction, and the subsequent daily struggles that followed these conditions, were also prominent subjects. Historically, jazz musicians, often of lower socioeconomic status, were predisposed to drug and alcohol addictions. Certainly these troubles influenced their lyrics, providing classist critics of the genre with plenty of low-hanging fruit to demonize jazz musicians with.

Increasingly, there was a mythos behind drugs and their seeming ability to improve the creative capacities of jazz players. Then, it may not come as a surprise that jazz musicians were on average eight times more likely to be drug dependent than the general population, and four times more likely to have a mood disorder. Perhaps, most damagingly, heroin reigned supreme as the most fashionable drug in the prominent jazz subgenre, bebop. It tended to increase the pleasure of playing and help artists come to terms with the downtrodden and bleak environments they operated in. This occupational stress, poor economic conditions, and mythology behind drugs perpetuated a cycle of mental illness and addiction within the jazz world.

Ultimately, some of the music served to glorify the drugs, but (often indirectly) denounce the fallout of the decisions to indulge such substances. The discourse of mental health within jazz didn't evolve far past this point. Given the limited awareness of mental health in the early 20th century and the socioeconomic problems that pervaded amongst jazz's prominent characters, this stunted discussion of mental illness isn't surprising.

Today, jazz is the canonical genre of musical academia given it's massive legacy and harmonic and rhythmic intricacies. Although the genre is preserved through this medium, it is much less relevant to pop culture and, by extension, the general population. As a result, the genre is not the site of controversy and cutting social discourse that it used to be.

Folk, Rock, and Things You Don't Discuss at the Dinner Table

Recommended Listens:

1. We shall Overcome (Live at Woodstock) - Joan Baez
2. This Land is Your Land - Woody guthrie
3. Hit Or Miss - Odetta
4. Tutti Frutti - Little Richard
5. The Times They Are A-Changin' - Bob Dylan
6. Revolution - The Beatles
7. Paint It, Black - The Rolling Stones
8. Soul Sacrifice (Live at The Woodstock Music & Art Fair, August 16, 1969) - Santana
9. My Generation - The Who
10. With A Little Help From My Friends - Joe Cocker
11. I Just Wasn't Made For These Times - The Beach Boys
12. Under Pressure - Queen, David Bowie

Since people have been questioning and rejecting the status quo, political music has existed. Music has been used to rebel as far back (and further even) as the French Revolution, and as recently as the ongoing Black Lives Matter movement of 2020 with songs like "Sweeter" by Leon Bridges or, in reference to the ongoing COVID-19 pandemic, songs like "In a Young Person's Body," in which Kora Feder sings, "'Cause our heroes are helpless and our leaders tell lies / Sometimes I wake up in the morning thinking everything's alright."

Protest songs express artists views on social and political injustice and often share the opinions of their audience. The Folk Revival, the British Invasion, and the Hippie Movement were all major American music movements that bled into each other throughout the 1950s to 1970s. They all impacted Western societies with their new ways of thinking and their rejection of war and oppression.

The Folk Revival throughout the United States produced artists like Woody Guthrie, The Weavers, the Almanac Brothers, and the founder of People's Songs, The Kingston Trio. These artists tended to be apolitical, but popularized folk and opened doors for artists like Joan Baez who was an activist in the civil rights movements, and my grandma Leslie's personal favourite, Odetta, known as "the queen of folk music."

During the 1950s, folk was driven underground for it's left-wing beliefs. However, this ostracization gave the genre a rebellious allure and only emboldened artists to spread more openly political messages. Many folk musicians played in the "coffee house circuit" for private parties that were often racially integrated and college-campus concerts. Their anthems, like "We Shall Overcome," which was performed at Martin Luther King's march in 1963 by various artists (Joan Baez, Pete Seeger, Josh White, Peter, Paul and Mary, and Bob Dylan), were messages of hope during the civil rights movement and played an important role in non-violent activism. These lyrics presented a promise of equality, such as the lines, "I do believe / We shall overcome, someday / We'll walk hand in hand, someday / We shall be free, someday / We shall live in peace, someday."

In the U.S., folk rock emerged from the Folk Music Revival and the influence that the Beatles and other British Invasion bands had on members of that movement. Folk rock is a hybrid music genre combining elements of folk music and rock music. Rock and roll had blasted out of the early fifties with the libidinal urgency only bestowed upon repressed teenagers. That is to say, rock and roll's origins did not reflect just how political the genre would become. Here, pure, primal feeling said it all, de-emphasizing the spotlight lyrics traditionally occupied in the minds of listeners. It was an explosive concoction blend of blues, jazz, and country, which instead highlighted the sounds of full-band instrumentation, the new invention of electric guitars, and emotional vocal inflection.

Then, it might not be too surprising that the lyrics of early rock and roll were close to being gibberish. Close, but not quite. Perhaps this early incarnation can be best summarized by Little Richard's unforgettable refrain in "Tutti Frutti," which reads as, "wop-bop-a-loo-mop alop-bom-boom." Clearly, such a well-composed lyric could be placed amongst the poetic greats like Keats and Frost.

 Rest-assured, these sorts of lyrics were largely about voraciously and vigorously expelling sexual urges; however, unlike the crooners who also sang about their passionate affairs, rock and roll transcended ethnic lines — an offensive notion to the puritan critics of the age. Ultimately, the gibberish of rock and roll was a necessary teen dialect which protected the music from loaded analysis.

But rock and roll changed headed into the 60s. Breaking from the boy-band-esque formula of the 50s which marketed artists to girls as objects of desire, the rock and roll bands of the 1960s served as the idols to young males who wanted to be just like them. So did the content of rock and roll change, and while eroticism remained a staple of the genre, so did social upheaval, much in response to the increasingly grim outlook of the Cold War and the impending asassination of the president John F. Kennedy. With these events came a more cynical and intense brand of young person, less concerned about being carefree, and more invested in political activism.

As a result, rock and roll music became integrally involved with movements for social change. American artists like Bob Dylan emerged, whose freedom songs ("Blowin' in the Wind," and "Times Are-a-Changin," amongst others) became anthems for both the Folk Revival and the Hippie Movement. At the same time, the themes of rock and roll music (and these social initiatives themselves) were embracing even more psychotropic drugs, casual sex, rebellion, women's rights, and differing interpretations of the "American Dream." Coinciding with the death of JFK, 1963 was a noticeable shift for rock and roll, and the music became more rebellious, depressing, and intellectually-challenging than before. The Vietnam War draft in 1969 only further exacerbated these trends, cementing the genre as the backdrop to anti-war sentiment and social commentary. This shift developed an anti-establishment cultural phenomenon amongst young people called the Counterculture movement, which advanced the Hippie Movement and the British Invasion.

Pop and rock musicians such as the Beatles, the Rolling Stones, the Who, the Kinks, the Dave Clark Five, Herman's Hermits, The Swinging Blue Jeans, the Zombies, and Dusty Springfield were at the forefront of the British Invasion. Many had openly political tunes. The Beatles' "Taxman," "Revolution," and "Blackbird," and The Rolling Stones' "We love you" and "Street Fighting Man" were amongst the top protest songs from the British Invasion. For example, the lyrics in "Revolution" state, "We all want to change the world / But when you talk about destruction / Don't you know that you can count me out." As the British music "invaded" the U.S., it intersected with this new wave thinking, creating a critical turning point in American history, and opening the floodgate for the Counterculture movement to fight the conservative lifestyles from the 1950s.

The Hippie Movement, also known as the Peace or Flower Power movement, further advanced the Counterculture way of thinking. Voices were raised from every gender and race asking for equality, freedom, and peace. This movement created an Expressivism view of life, where a quest for self-expression by grooving on or getting into music and art, psychedelic drugs, concern for others, affiliation, religious, philosophical, and spiritual interests became the popular interest among young people of America. One of the important roles the Hippies had was popularizing non-violent protests and activism, and music was at the center of this. There were three main events that solidified the Hippie movement.

The first was the "Human Be-In" event in 1970 in San Francisco, held at the Golden Gate Park and attended by approximately 30,000 hippies. It was here that Timothy Leary, a writer and psychologist, coined the now-famous line, "Turn up, Tune in, Drop out," by which he meant to become more sensitive to your consciousness, interact harmoniously with the world around you, and commit to choice and change. This phrase helped shape the entire hippie counterculture, as it voiced the key ideas of 1960s rebellion.

The second event was called the "Summer of Love" and lasted from June to October 1967, where hippies convened in most major cities in America, Canada, and Europe, but most notably in the Haight-Ashbury District, San Francisco. San Francisco's participants alone are predicted to have been around 100,000 people, and was the cultural center of the Hippie movement where free love, drug use, and communal living became the norm. This period of time also helped spawn the widespread "flower children" that became a major American symbol in the 1960s because of their idealistic views, and are synonymous with the term "hippie."

The third event that the Hippie movement — with all it's peaceful protests, groovy music, and liberal beliefs — was leading up to was in August of 1969. Woodstock: "3 Days of Peace and Music" was a four day music and arts festival that took place on a rural dairy farm in New York State, attracting a crowd of 400,000 people. This event was the culmination of years of social experimentation and changing social practices, resulting in an event like none-other. Many of the attendees of the festival said their goal was to demonstrate that if they could have that many people together with absolutely no violence, then they could bring that love back into society. They believed they could change the world. And they did. What started with a capitalist idea to make revenue ended up making no profit and resulted in a drastic change to America's reality. In the words of Max Yasgur, who owned the dairy farm those young hippies occupied, they have "proven to this world a half a million young people can get together and have three days of fun and music, and have nothing but fun and music! And God bless [them] for it."

The artists that performed during the historical four days were the voices of change that these "young hippies" looked up to. Richie Havens kicked off the first day after arriving before any other artists including his own bandmates. He informed the organizers that there were so many people blocking traffic to get to this festival that there was no way the artists would be arriving anywhere close to on time, so they ended up flying the artists in via helicopter. Meanwhile, Havens played for nearly 2 full hours. He ended his show by singing "Freedom," a song he wrote in that very moment that would become the anthem of Woodstock. Other notable performances were "Soul Sacrificed" by Santana, "Higher" by Sly & the Family Stone, "My Generation" by The Who, "Sunday Morning" by Jefferson Airplane, "A Little Help from Friends" by Joe Cocker, "Suite: Judy Blue Eyes" by Crosby, Stills, & Nash, and finally the USA National Anthem turned imitation of war by Jimmy Hendrix labeled as a "quintessential piece of art." All of these artists and many more sang out in peaceful protest, influencing generations to come.

While Protest songs pathed the way for open dialogue on an expansive range of topics, one issue they rarely touched on was mental health. Political music, especially related to the Hippie Era, often discussed the idea of opening your mind beyond your preconceived notions but failed to make connections to genuine mental health problems.

There are exceptions to the rule that we should acknowledge. With the tidal shift of lyrical content in rock and roll came a small wellspring of songs that addressed mental health issues like addiction, loneliness, and depression. The Rolling Stones' classic, "Paint It, Black," strongly represents this rock and roll's shift to darker topics, addressing death, depression, and social nihilism in their skepticism of the status-quo. The track is a stark departure from the bubblegum-esque rock and roll of the 1950s.

In similar light, Brian Wilson of the Beach Boys chronicled his struggles with depression and his impending mental breakdown in the 1966 song, "I Just Wasn't Made For These Times," which concerned his growing feelings of isolation. It is a noticeable display of vulnerability for a band most well known for peppy jams and sun-soaked barber-shop harmonies.

While the mental health discourse in rock and roll continued to be overshadowed by it's more culturally-relevant themes as it moved forward into the future, some songs continued to push boundaries. One great example is the song, "Under Pressure," penned by Queen and David Bowie. The passage, "It's the terror of knowing what the world is about / Watching some good friends screaming 'let me out,'" acknowledges the growing cynicism and existential dread of time, while empathizing with those grappling with suicidal thoughts. Ultimately, "Under Pressure" is a shining example of what a song concerning mental health issues can be. Rock and roll and protest music at large may not be known for inciting a wave of mental health awareness, but it contains some great early examples of the impact music could have on these topics.

Soda and All That Other Fizz

Recommended Listens:

1. Love Shack - The B-52's
2. Billie Jean - Michael Jackson
3. Kiss - Prince
4. I Wanna Dance With Somebody (Who Loves Me) - Whitney Houston
5. As Long As You Love Me - The Backstreet Boys
6. Wannabe - Spice Girls
7. Telephone - Lady Gaga, Beyonce
8. Stronger (What Doesn't Kill You) - Kelly Clarkson
9. Señorita - Shawn Mendes, Camila Cabello
10. Girl Can Rock - Hilary Duff
11. Keep Holding On - Avril Lavigne
12. Sk8er Boi - Avril Lavigne

What do you think of when you envision pop music?

Teenagers in neon, moonwalking around to Micheal Jackson's latest hits? Screaming adolescence girls throwing themselves over guardrails to get a better glance at the totally cute boy band, NSYNC? Or maybe the fishnet fingerless gloves and bangles look inspired by the goddess herself, Avril Lavigne?

Whatever you picture, you remember the lyrics, the poppy beat, and unstoppable urge to sing along. Whatever era, pop music made its way into our hearts and brains — playing over and over and over … and over again.

The term "pop" may refer to several different definitions. For example, the New Grove Dictionary of Music and Musicians describes popular music as what was most widely accepted in the urban middle class since the industrialization period. However, this definition is too broad for any meaningful analysis, as hundreds of genres with both similar and contradictory sonic qualities climbed to the top of Billboard's Hot 100 throughout the years.

Consequently, this chapter focuses on the lineage of pop that evolved from rock and roll, featuring catchy hooks, danceable beats, and the latest recording technology and production techniques. The New Grove Dictionary of Music and Musicians claims that the term "pop music" originated during the mid-1950s in Britain to broadly describe "non-classical music" that influences new youth music styles. In the 1960s, pop music's definition was narrowed by being categorized as beat music overlapped with rock n roll.

This chapter further narrows its focus by beginning with pop music from the 1980s. The rationale is that pop music in decades past was essentially synonymous with rock and roll music. For example, bands that were considered pop music in the 1960s and 1970s like The Beatles, Rolling Stones, Led Zeppelin, and David Bowie are also known as rock and roll royalty. Even artists like Elton John and the Jackson 5 retained rock elements in their instrumentation. However, the 80s saw a sharp turn into beat instrumentation through mixing technology instead of rock and roll standards like electric guitar, bass, and acoustic drums.

Pop music extends across all walks a life. The man in the business suit? He knows the lyrics to "Love Shack" from front to back. The mom dropping off her kids at school? She's got Lady Gaga blasting on the radio. Your neighbour down the street just downloaded Post Malone's newest single. The reason why pop music seems to attract such a massive audience is because it continuously takes influence from other genres. Genres like rock, punk, R&B, and hip-hop have all been amalgamated into pop over at some point. We can hear these fusions with artists like Ed Sheeran (who has an entire Collaborations Project album), Kelly Clarkson, Drake, and Beyonce. Other genres, like Latin, have started making appearances in the last ten years with artists like Shawn Mendes, Camila Cabello, and Enrique Iglesias.

While this genre seems to take hold of so many genre styles, the lyrics behind the songs seem to go in the same direction - love and having fun.

Some of the most prevalent pop artists in the 1980s almost solely wrote about love. "Billie Jean," by Micheal Jackson, is about getting a pretty girl pregnant. "Kiss," by Prince, is about wooing a girl into kissing you. Almost every single one of Whitney Houston's hits are about being in love including "I Wanna Dance With Somebody," "How Will I Know," and "Saving All My Love For You." Radio bumped these tunes 24/7, every walkman had a CD, and every teen awkwardly slow-danced to them at homecoming.

There are exceptions. Madonna's hit "Material Girl" can be interpreted as an extension of the feminist movement; however, ultimately the image of many pop songs in 80s were completely wrapped around the idea of heteronormative relationships. This era's particular conformity to the stereotypical love ballads could be because of the lack of diversity at the time in the pop genre. A London based research team actually found that American mainstream music has a great amount of sonic variation except for one decade: the 80s. During this time, 71% of all pop lyrical content was about love and relationships and the instrumentals were restricted to either full on dance pop or hard rock.

In a generation obsessed with being "cool" (as quoted by my mother-in-law and proven in George Michael's music video, "Father Figure"), it is possible this narrow narrative surrounding love was damaging for the young people listening. There are many groups and minorities that seem to be left out of the conversation such as the mentally ill or LGBTQ community. Does that mean they are destined to be alone forever? Of course not, but to a young impressionable mind, they might think so.

The lyrical trends of the 80s more or less persisted moving forward into the next decade, albeit with some small yet significant changes. Artists like Backstreet Boys, Spice Girls, NSYNC, and Aqua blended love songs with dance party beats. Moody love ballads were slowly phased out, conceding to the increasingly popular bouncy love songs that included the idea of having fun (insert glitter bomb here). Songs about partying and having a good time jumped from 4% to 10% in the 90s.

Love still comprised the majority of pop music in this decade, pervading in 66% of all Billboard charting singles. On that note, the 90s is particularly noticeable for the emergence of boy bands and girl groups directed specifically towards young teenagers. The Backstreet Boys track, "As Long As You Love Me," features a dramatic chorus about being so desperate for love that it did not even matter who the girl was. A similar pattern is evident in songs like "Say You'll Be There" by the Spice Girls. The pop hit depicts a person willing to dedicate every ounce of themselves to someone without expecting any reciprocation.

The question then becomes whether it is damaging that the canonical genre of Western culture continuously depicts a single perspective on love. Many of these conceptions of relationships are unbalanced and set unrealistic and unsustainable standards for the way a loving relationship should operate. Since these pop artists are almost solely listened to by young impressionable girls, the lyrical content can be problematic for how they develop future relationships and potentially damage their self-esteem and mental health.

In a (shockingly long, 12-hour) interview, the late rock and roll legend Frank Zappa posits that the "love lyrics" craze in pop music contributes to poor mental health in America. In his view, these types of lyrics create an illusion of what relationships should be, but can actually never be achieved. The songwriters are creating a facade of personal turmoil that creates a protocol for how you should behave in a romantic relationship. Children growing up listening to these lyrics about fairytale relationships and melodramatic breakups are building false depictions of love. These lyrical tendencies essentially create a group of "love loser[s]" who are forever searching for something that does not exist. This mentality is toxic and correlates with declining mental health.

These songs are not just romantic serenades being sung in front of a sunset and candlelight dinner. Many are degrading songs about how people (mostly women) should be willing to sacrifice anything for their partner under the banner of love. Frank Zappa's take on this issue is especially compelling given his success in the music industry and his experience with the top of the Billboard charts. Consequently, Zappa knew what artists and songwriters were willing to do to make a profit and gain a massive fan base.

It could be possible that the prevalence of these types of songs leave less room for the discourse of mental health in pop music. For example, one study that analyzed lyrical content in pop music found an extremely low frequency of songs containing any references to depression and suicide throughout the 80s, 90s, and early 2000s. Shockingly, no mainstream pop songs in the 80s contain any references. This trend changed slightly to 1% in the 90s but then regressed to 0.8% in the early 2000s.

The pop music of the early 2000s was split in terms of intended audiences, caught between the worlds of teenage pop and adult contemporary. Artists like Hilary Duff sang about growing up and rites of passage, as opposed to artists like Christina Aguilera, who belted about throwing down in the club. Still, the concept of love was relatively high in pop lyrics, making up 64.6% of songs. Interestingly, tracks about dancing and having fun skyrocketed to 39.6% compared to the 19% in the 80s.

While lyrics about depression and suicide dipped to 0.8%, there is a unique case of one singer that defined her brand around issues tangential or directly about mental health. That singer is Avril Lavigne. Tellingly, she had not one but six songs that reflected the struggles that accompany depression in her first three studio albums. Songs like "I'm With You" and "Tomorrow" seem to be personal experiences or at least told in first person context. The lyrics somberly address the experience of loneliness rather than present it as a symptom of not being in a Hollywood-esque relationship.

This approach contradicts so much of pop music wherein the protagonist of the lyrics, typically a woman, wishes for a significant other to whisk them away from feelings of isolation. Even Avril Lavigne has her fair share of these types of tracks; still, these other chart-topping songs are truly innovative in their discourse of mental health, addressing the isolation and perpetual emptiness which is inherent in depression. "Keep Holding On" is about supporting someone with mental illness and encouraging those to keep moving through life even when it gets difficult.

So why was this teen singer so revolutionary when it came to mental health?

One possible explanation is that Avril Lavigne was drawing from different sonic and lyrical influences than many of her contemporaries: the "emo" scene — a grassroots descendant of punk rock which had recently exploded into the mainstream consciousness during the 2000s. Emo music was infamous, and at the time, maligned, for its unabashed focus on just what the name implied: emotion. In the fourth part of this book, we will return to pop's relationship with mental illness to see how, after the mainstream rise of third wave emo, pop began addressing mental illness on a much wider scale.

PART TWO: CHEER UP, EMO KID

First Wave: Softboiled Hardcore Toughguys

Recommended Listens:

1. Anarchy in the U.K. - Sex Pistols
2. Blitzkrieg Bop - Ramones
3. Train in Vain (Stand by Me) - The Clash
4. United Blood - Agnostic Font
5. No One Rules - Agnostic Font
6. Deeper Than Inside - Rites of Spring
7. Theme - Rites of Spring
8. Guilty of Being White - Minor Threat
9. White Minority - Black Flag
10. Said Gun - Embrace
11. No More Pain - Embrace

As we have attempted to demonstrate in part one, mental health has been periodically addressed across various styles and music. However, these references and disclosures tend to be the exception, not the rule. Conversely, topics surrounding mental health comprise the foundation of the current wave of "emo" music.

Before emo, there was punk rock, which emerged in the mid-1970s in the hallowed halls of the legendary New York club, CBGB's. Contrary to the overproduced and increasingly complex mainstream rock, punk emphasized simplicity, anti-commercialism, and authenticity. These characteristics empowered young people who lacked the means to develop the musical prowess necessary for the era's popular music. However, this sort of appeal ultimately didn't resonate with the affluent and prosperous American population of the time, and the music did not achieve great cultural relevance. Sorry, punk rock, America can't hear you through all your poor.

It would be a different story a few years later during the UK's economic recession. Here, the ease of which punk music could be played made it accessible to charismatic personalities who had an anti-establishment message to spread to a down-trodden populace. It was like glycerine set ablaze. Punk exploded with bands like the Sex Pistols, the Ramones, and The Clash charging into the forefront of pop culture. In turn, the craze finally infected America airwaves in a big way. This wave of punk rock was relatively short-lived, with many music scholars citing 1979 as the end, neatly correlating with prominent punk frontman Sid Vicious' death and Margaret Thatcher's onset Conservative takeover of the UK government.

With the implosion of punk came several diverging genres that took influence, such as Oi!, street punk, and, most prominently, hardcore. Unlike punk, hardcore was primarily regulated to America's East coast at first. While toughness, political messages, and fast tempos were emphasized in punk, hardcore took these characteristics to their extremes. The music was extremely aggressive, capitalizing on emotions of anger, frustration, and upset. A show could just as quickly spur a ferocious brawl as it could a mosh pit, attracting an extremely dedicated, hyper-masculine fan base. Not quite Chads, but definitely Jakes.

By 1985, hardcore had taken over east and west coast underground music venues; the violent, enraged, and political hardcore bands and fans were raving, rioting, moshing, and mobbing all across America, Canada, and the United Kingdom.

In New York particularly, an influx of hardcore bands, such as Cro Mags, Agnostic Front, and Warzone, were tearing up underground venues with vicious, angry, politically charged anthems for disgruntled youth in the unforgiving city.

In early February, a few leagues south of the hardcore capital, in the capital of the country, Washington, D.C., a band named Rites of Spring, had just entered the recording studio for the first time. This new band, formed by Guy Picciotto, Michael Fellows, Brendan Canty, and Eddie Janney, were about to make their first and last record under an independent record label named Dischord. The label was run by other founding members of the Washington scene, such as Ian MacKaye, the vocalist for a major hardcore punk band — Minor Threat.

Rites of Spring became leaders in the Revolution Summer of 1985. A movement in punk politics that challenged the stereotypical punk image of a tough guy raging at the capitalist machine with mosh pit beatdowns and masculine anger. Despite it's spread across the States, hardcore had remained a relatively niche genre. Hitting a ceiling imposed by the political and Fight Club-esque qualities of its music scene, which alienated newcomers, some punks, and artists alike. Recognizing these limits, the Revolution Summer was searching for new punk politics that were more inclusive and sensitive.

The Revolution Summer was a conversation within the hardcore scene on the purpose, direction, and future of the genre. Leading artists and up and comers discussed ways to evolve their art and began experimenting with personal lyrics that offered an image of a broken, emotional, and despairing heart, rather than one raging with hatred and macho man politics. It also perfectly coincides with the June release of the self-titled Rites of Spring.

Rites of Spring is often considered one of the first emocore or emo albums in existence due to its confessional and desperately honest lyrics. They also took the classic aggressive punk and hardcore sounds that were popular and fused them with melodic guitar lines to open up new possibilities in emotional expression that wasn't available to the chromatic or minor key power chords that characterized hardcore and punk.

The lyrical topics of emocore still circulated anti-establishment political issues, but extended far beyond that, discussing social alienation and romantic relationships. Ian MacKaye, the frontman of Embrace, was also a champion of the straight edge ideology, whose pious followers abstained from some combination of alcohol, drugs, and sex.

An example will show the drastic change between lyrical content that made Rites of Spring stand out as a new act in town. Agnostic Front, leaders in the hardcore scene, lyrically enforced their aggressive punk politics which had a "you're either in or you're out" mentality toward rebelling against authority and staying loyal to the punk scene.

For example, the song "United Blood" demands a high standard of its audience to partake in the punk community actively: "Talk about unity, talk about conformity / You don't want to support the scene / Why don't you get the fuck away from me." The song, "No One Rules" combines vulgarity and war-like seriousness to assert their point: "You got no right to tell us what to do / You got no balls to tell us what to do / There ain't no joke and there's no fuckin' break." The former lyric offers up a tough-guy image of a man ready to fight for his music, while aggressively calling out hardcore imposters.

The latter is a masculine rebellion against the American government and the mainstream culture of the 1980s.

On the other hand, on the album, Rites of Spring, we find songs such as "Deeper Than Inside," an introspective track zoning in on internal sorrow, exploring the heretofore unexplored topic of emotions, stating: "And you wonder / just how lost inside can be? / Try me, try me." We also hear confessional tunes like "Theme" admitting to considerable pain and unbearable despair: "And hope is just another rope / to hang myself with / to tie me down." On this song we also find vocalist, Guy Picciotto, challenging the listener to open a line to their emotions, asking, "And if I started crying, / Would you start crying? / Now I started crying / Why are you not crying?" To answer the question, yes I am crying.

Another Revolution Summer band, Embrace, followed similar lyrical motifs. Embrace was fronted by Ian Mackaye, the lead vocalist of Minor Threat, who had signed Rites of Spring to his independent label. As part of the emotional hardcore uprising, MacKaye moved away from his provocative (and frankly inappropriate in today's world) political and cacophonous lyrics. They expressed anger and hatred at the world around him and channeled personal feelings and insights into melodies that, though aggressively shouted, would become stock in every emo band.

We can easily see and hear the difference between MacKaye's pre-revolution Minor Threat themes and the musical content of Embrace's 1985 summer arrival. Embrace's first and only album, self-titled Embrace, was released in 1987 but written during the hotbed of the Revolution Summer. Minor Threat lyrics contain many political ideas and aggressively confront civil rights trends emerging in the mainstream. For example, "Guilty of Being White" complains about the academic and layman pursuits for slavery reparations, claiming "I'm sorry / For something that I didn't do / Lynched somebody / But I don't know who / You blame me for slavery / A hundred years before I was born."

To be fair to the punks, these ignorant themes weren't accepted across the board. Bands like Black Flag had songs like "White Minority" (released in 1981) which had already made fun of immature gripes like MacKaye's, trying to depict such a thinker as outrageous and absurd.

However, even MacKaye quickly switched gears away from controversial topics to address social issues more uniquely and productively. First, songs like "Said Gun" gave a more empathetic view of MacKaye as he looked critically on his scene: "Look what you've organized / Do you believe all those lies / There's no courage in hatred / Only in love / Look what you've organized." He seems to criticize the hatred and lack of empathy present in traditional punk in favor of an open, loving community.

More importantly, Embrace began speaking on emo themes, explicitly addressing mental health issues. "No More Pain" fits this bill, closing with the following:

> "No more tough-guy stance
> I hear your mommy call
> No more suicide
> It kills everyone
> No more petty love
> No more petty hate
> No more pettiness
> No more pain"

Here MacKaye explicitly faces the both the macho-man attitude and the consequences on men's abilities to share their mental health problems. The song suggests that we need to address the masculine bravado that pretends their unending anger and aggression is not a sign of poor mental health. The refusal to admit a soft side has allowed the hardcore scene to drink the "Kool-aid" (a reference to the Jonestown massacre) propaganda that drugs and alcohol are valid responses to the pain they feel. Thus, MacKaye sings on "Said Gun:" "There's no courage in hatred / Only in love."

The Revolution Summer brought on the use of the term "emo" to describe the new wave of emotional hardcore that was arising. This first wave of emo was not going to be the last, and would not compare to the tsunamis of the upcoming emo surges.

Second Wave: We Like Choruses Now

Recommended Listens:

1. Lithium - Nirvana
2. Grendel - Sunny Day Real Estate
3. Black Hole Sun - Soundgarden
4. Puddle Splashers - Cap'n Jazz
5. The Middle - Jimmy Eat World
6. Vengance Factor - Further Seems Forever

Despite its more inclusive values, emocore arguably was more a niche in hardcore for the remainder of the 1980s. It wasn't until the next decade that the needle would begin to pick up. The stratospheric rise of Nirvana and grunge would soon change that. Influenced by hardcore and punk, grunge erased the overproduced and shallow glam rock as the most popular form of rock music seemingly overnight. This takeover shifted the general populace's music palettes to embrace rawer sounds and lyrics about dejection, teenage angst, and sadness. The shift set the stage for the next wave of emo bands to attract more attention, given their sonic and ideological similarities with grunge.

By the time second-wave emo appeared in the scene in its fullfledged form in the mid to late 90s, the genre had expanded and developed a considerable amount. Second wave emo continued with confessional-style lyrics that confronted introspective personal problems while further evolving aspects of sound to create more delineated emo. Taking the aggression of emocore and amplifying the nascent singing styles and melodies, the second wave, or

Midwest emo, used the loud, distorted guitars, dirty bass tones, and explosive drum kits to create heartfelt and somber songs. Yet this time around, the songs were catchy.

No longer designed to tear down the establishment and its musical standards, the second wave of emo was more willing to use mainstream techniques. The techniques included in-key catchy and melodic vocals or traditional rock song structures. The second-wave emo gained more traction amongst a broader and larger audience by incorporating these aspects of 90s alt-rock, grunge, and pop-punk. We could say the second wave ran with the business model: "Pained Hearts; Pleased Ears."

For all these reasons, these bands tended to be much more accessible to the audiences of the 1990s. They began to amass a much larger following, such as Sunny Day Real Estate, who had the added benefit of being labelmates with Nirvana and Soundgarden. And while grunge mostly died out in 1994 with the tragic death of Nirvana vocalist Kurt Cobain, emo continued to thrive as an active underground music scene.

Lyrical content remained similar to the old emocore and touched on topics of mental health, despair, anger, and depression indirectly through sound and metaphor particularly.

A prime example of this indirect conversation about mental health comes from the song "Grendel" by Sunny Day Real Estate. The band is widely considered quintessential emo. Their album featuring "Grendel" titled Diary, is required reading for anyone wondering what emo is all about. "Grendel" only consists of three lines, which refer to a great deal of sadness and isolation: "The rain was there to wash away my tears / I wanted to be them, but instead I destroyed my chance / Suede scars." However, via the title, the song refers to the Old English epic poem, Beowulf. The narrator of "Grendel" compares the sadness of marginalization to the feeling that the monstrous antagonist, Grendel, experiences Beowulf's experiences. Like Grendel, the narrator feels like a community is hunting him, that he is a monster, and that his destruction is imminent and deserved. The song may be providing a sympathetic reading to the monster of Beowulf. Yet, it may, on the other hand, be providing a self-deprecating reading of the narrator. Either way, the melancholy guitar lines, the friendship with rain, and the desire to be someone else all fill the song with depressing and vulnerable undertones.

The album, Diary, is a great title depicting the newfound world of lyrical content that artists would begin to pursue: a world of introspection, teenage angst, and emotional expression. In one way or another, each emo song would feel like a page ripped from a teenage diary. Raw, honest, often ugly, and upset, emo became a place for audiences and artists alike to outlet emotions they felt were not addressed in the regular world.

Cap'n Jazz was another midwest second-wave emo band to take on angst and woe in a melodic yet aggressive style. They also, like most of the other fundamental and genre-defining bands we've mentioned, only had one album, which was jokingly titled: Burritos, Inspiration Point, Fork Balloon Sports, Cards in the Spokes, Automatic Biographies, Kites, Kung Fu, Trophies, Banana Peels We've Slipped On and Egg Shells We've Tippy Toed Over.

Cap'n Jazz took the intense emotional expression and placed within witty rhymes and bitter-sweet nostalgia. The title of one song, "Puddle Splashers," gives the listener a snapshot of children playing in rainwater puddles. Even still, through nostalgic memories, Cap'n Jazz managed to encapsulate the emo-defining desperation within intense instrumentals and exposed lyrics: "I remember her saying / 'This whole world is a waste of my time' / All I could say is / 'I wish I had something to say.'" The narrator reflects on memories and the profound impact they've had on his development. He points to an unidentified person's critical and common feeling of depression, "the world is a waste of my time." He recognizes the sincerity of this person's declaration and seems to have a close connection to them since he begs, "hold me here dearest and turn me gold." The narrator regards this unnamed person highly and can see that, though "I watched you holding up the sun," darkness hangs over their head. "I wish I had something to say," laments the speaker, wishing the right words to address such sorrow would come to mind.

Indeed, second-wave emo was able to recognize mental health problems implicitly through the topics they addressed. However, mental health had yet to be at the forefront of discussion. This absence would soon change.

A crystallizing moment for emo came in 1997 when Deep Elm Records began to release a compilation series known as the Emo Diaries. Until this time, emo had mostly been a niche term, often confused with hardcore or indie rock. Now, the genre's independence would be enshrined in the minds of alternative music fans, primarily because the series featured several breakout acts, such as Jimmy Eat World and Further Seems Forever. Armed with more even pop sensibilities and polished production than their predecessors, these bands took their sound to mainstream audiences. By the early 2000s, the term "emo" was being discussed in popular magazines such as Rolling Stone, Alternative Press, and Seventeen Magazine.

Finally, after years of the vague term "emo" floating around hardcore punks to college campuses, the name hit the mainstream in a particular form: kids expressing their mental health in an overt, loud, and aggressive way. It was the beginning of emo's third and most well-known wave. This incarnation of emo would become so popular in the mid-2000s; it would be known as a mainstream subculture.

Third Wave: The Coolest Losers in the World

Recommended Listens:

1. Note To Self - From First to Last
2. Hold On - Good Charlotte
3. Understanding in a Car Crash - Thursday
4. I'm Not Okay (I promise) - My Chemical Romance
5. 7 Minutes In Heaven (Atavan Halen) - Fall Out Boy
6. Face Down - The Red Jumpsuit Apparatus
7. Nothing to Lose - Billy Talent
8. Irony of Dying on Your Birthday - Senses Fail
9. Family Tradition - Senses Fail
10. Modern Chemistry - Motion City Soundtrack
11. The Church Channel - Say Anything
12. I Don't Feel Very Receptive Today - Underoath
13. To Plant a Seed - We Came As Romans

Ironically, as emo became a defined movement in the mainstream consciousness, emo's sound was becoming more difficult to pinpoint. Post-hardcore acts like From First to Last and From Autumn to Ashes were considered emo. Metalcore bands like Underoath and 18 visions were emo. So were pop-punk artists like Good Charlotte and Fall Out Boy. More head-scratching variants of the genre included folk (ala Bright Eyes) and 80s New Wave Throwbacks (Nightmare of You).

These artists were loosely grouped because of their emotional lyrical content, but more prominently because of their fashion. As the 2000s progressed, emo became synonymous with a fashion amalgamation of several underground 90s music scenes. T-shirts, black-rimmed glasses, long hair from 90s indie rock met tropes from goth and punk subcultures, such as black and neon colours, skinny jeans, and macabre imagery. Gender-bending was also characteristic of this look, with eyeliner and black nail polish becoming trademarks of emo.

Evidently, third-wave emo is so massive, complex, undefined, and unexplained that making a claim such as: "emo music dealt primarily with mental health" or "a lyrical focus on teenage angst characterizes emo" is pointless. Emo bands, like any other skilled artist, write a variety of songs and albums with a variety of sounds, themes, instruments, and lyrics. However, bands began to write more and more individual songs related to mental health than ever before. Further, since part of the emo style is honest, unadulterated personal feeling, emo writers with mental health issues consistently wrote songs about mental health, which ranged from insightful and relatable to disturbing and concern-raising. Examining how emo music brought mental health to the centre stage will require examples from emo bands, both household names and underground legends.

Thursday was an early example of the emo genre taking a deep dive into mental health and its related topics. The song "Dying in New Brunswick" off of their first full-length album, Waiting, contains a voyeuristic look at the opening statement in a personal letter from a desperate narrator to an unknown addressee: "I'm writing you this letter to let you know that I'm not alright." The first song after the intro on their second full-length album, Full Collapse, titled "Understanding in a Car Crash," attempts to capture the post-traumatic experience for the survivor of a car crash. In this track, like a direct response to his initial letter an album before, addresses the unknown listener, "I don't wanna feel this way forever / a dead letter marked 'return to sender.'"

An example of a household name, My Chemical Romance, also became capstone archetypal emo role models, rocking edgy haircuts, black eyeliner, straightened hair, and jeans tighter than an aerospace airlock. As was the trend since emo began, Gerard Way, the frontman of the band, rejected the notion that his band was emo... but that has always been just as much a sign of ironic emo self-deprecation as it has been a sign of an honest remark. Their music combined punk, metal, and pop (along with heavy influences of swing and jazz) to create rockish sounding music. However, that music was filled with screaming, angst, tortured lovers, and intense emotional expression.

Way tended to write concept albums about tragic events, such as a Bonnie and Clyde style romance. Still, individual songs were taken by fans to mean something incredibly different from the original story Way presented. There is also a chance that Way knew his songs looked and sounded emo, and allowed for a double meaning to develop. Either way, a song like "I'm Not Okay (I Promise)," where the chorus repeats the words "I'm not okay," instantly became an emo anthem that resonated with the youth, especially the mentally ill.

Stigma surrounding mental health was still rampant in the 90s and early 2000s. So, having a group of young misfits bringing awareness to such a taboo subject was pretty revolutionary. Many bands in the scene were open about their personal experiences with bullying, suicide, trauma, grief, and mental illness. Fall Out Boy has always kept audiences listening for their complex and witty metaphors hiding meaning behind the music. The frontman, Pete Wentz, was open about his struggles with his undiagnosed bipolar disorder during his early career and his suicide attempt in 2005. This confession is a massive topic that most people would be uncomfortable admitting, but accessibility through music made a safe place for people experiencing the same conflict.

Wentz eventually became an international superstar, so his mental health struggles were frontpage headlines imprinted in the minds of his young fan base. They saw him as an exemplary role model, a lasting legend bravely facing mental illness. He captured the mindset behind his attempted suicide, related to his overwhelming stardom, commitments, young adult drama, and mental illness, in the song "7 Minutes in Heaven (Atavan Halen)," which ties together the Atavan Wentz overdosed on, and their rockstar fame (referencing Van Halen). Wentz portrays the connection between his mental illness and suicide attempt in two revealing lines: "I'm having another episode / I just need a stronger dose."

Once 3rd wave emo exploded, it became present across all hemispheres; and the topics it addressed, namely poor mental health and its various causes and effects, appeared in every band in the scene. It would be impossible to list them all. However, noteworthy hits include "Face Down" by Red Jumpsuit Apparatus, which condemns domestic abuse, and "Nothing to Lose" by Billy Talent, which tells the story of a high-school kid's suicide from the victim's perspective.

 Some bands made mental health topics their primary focus. Senses Fail's first album, Let it Enfold You, reads like a diary of angry and depressing thoughts, completed through a shaky singing voice and despairing, cry-like screams that immediately bring an uncontrollable meltdown and eruption of emotions to mind (see the first 35-45 seconds of "Irony of Dying on Your Birthday"). On their second album, Still Searching, the song "Sick or Sane (Fifty for a Twenty)" contains the lines: "Am I a little sick, or a little sane? / Cause I feel a little sick." Finally, their third album, Life is Not a Waiting Room, contains the song "Family Tradition," which discusses the genetic influences on the singer, Buddy Nielsen's, depression and addiction problems. The chorus runs as follows: "So, help me / Please, someone, come quick / I think I am losing it / Forgive me, I inherited this / From a stranger I'll never miss / I'm sick." Bands like Senses Fail embraced an unfiltered, unfettered, and brutally honest expression of raw emotions related to mental health experiences.

Some other bands took from second-wave emo and preferred

a more indirect approach, disguising mental health within fun-sounding songs, yet, unlike the second wave, explicitly addressing mental health without metaphor. Motion City Soundtrack was such a band. They dressed in a nerdier outfit, making them less of a niche band for rebellious teens who wanted to sound edgy and look "scene" (to be fair, the lead singer, Justin Pierre, did have an eclectic and recognizable look). In their catchy, Moog synthesizer pop-punk, which they marketed to a wide range of listeners, they addressed anxiety and depression in many songs, such as "Everything is Alright," "A-OK," and "Modern Chemistry." The latter explicitly addresses Pierre's struggles with anxiety, OCD, and alcoholism and describes it clearly in plain language: "They say I suffer from a lack of serotonin / Synapses they happen too / Infrequently for me / To be functioning properly." The chorus contains the following "nursery rhyme" that Pierre sarcastically sings:

> "I believe in medication
> And I believe in therapy
> And I believe in Crystal Light
> Cause I believe in me, yeah
> It's so uplifting, fuck yeah"

The nursery rhyme is one that therapists would drill into a mentally ill person's head. However, Pierre tells us, "I took the pills, I took the advice / The panic stopped, but still, I'm not right." In other words, though Pierre moved in the right direction by addressing his mental health issues and taking the proper medication, he still has not addressed the root cause. Thus, when he's "barely off the medication ... the walls are closing in again." Pierre knows the importance of facing his mental health issues and wants to get better, but lacks for some reason or another. In particular, we can see that the medical system has, in some way, let him down, whether a lousy doctor, underdeveloped medication, or something else. Whatever the exact cause, he still has reached the point of trusting the medical world to help his illness properly.

Perhaps the most extreme example of artists discussing mental illness openly in third-wave emo is the band Say Anything. Frontman, Max Bemis, dealt with bipolar disorder and struggled with self-medication and addiction issues for a long time. The song "Church Channel" describes Bemis falling in love in the psych ward after experiencing a psychotic break during the recording of the first Say Anything album, ...Is a Real Boy. He tells us, "I wake up in a room and realize I'm insane again," and since entering the hospital, "I fell behind on my nightly four-course meal of rainbow pills." Already, we have a bleak and explicit depiction of mental health and the inertia of medication and segregation from the public.

However, he meets a "ghost who keeps walking by my door," a girl that is also in treatment. She identifies with Bemis because he understands the stigma of mental illness "Oh, do you remember me? / Is your mind that worn? / We both were born / To be one with that which the public scorned." Even though the outside world despises the two lovers, they find solace in each other, repeating each other over and over at the end of the song, "So lay your head on me / So lay your head onto me."

Bemis also addresses the song "Sorry, Dudes, My Bad" to his band mates who had to manage touring with Bemis during his self-medicating addiction. He opens up with an honest cry for help:

> "It's too much to do on my own
> My friends, I need you now
> I'm sorry that I wrecked that tour for us
> The drugs left me wigging out on the bus"

Bemis began combating mental health stigma by writing about their emotional effects, which happened to connect with an audience of emo kids who shared similar experiences. Bemis helped start the next emo wave, which addressed the need for support and professional treatment, with his open discussions about his mental illness and addiction problems that didn't glorify the illness.

Now, another exciting thing happened in third-wave emo, which we talked about earlier in this section, that ended up changing the scope of emo once and for all. What happened is that people, including emos, labelled everything emotional, confessional, and dramatic "emo." This change meant that other genres, which were never before considered emo proper and aggressively opposed to emo, were subsumed under the same name. Punk, punk-rock, pop-punk, hardcore, post-hardcore, metal, metalcore, rock, and indie all had the potential to become emo based on their specific content. Form and genre started to become meaningless to the definition of "emo" since they only helped differentiate the music's sound, not necessarily the lyrical and emotional content of the piece, which were the real determining factor on whether something was emo or not.

This unification meant that all types of mental health issues, which were especially considered emo topics, could be expressed in various forms, including ones more fitting to encapsulate their reality. To explore this a little bit, we'll take a look at some more examples.

As our introduction mentions, the goal in this book is to talk about the emo music scene as it relates to mental health, so our explanations of different genres and subgenres have and will remain relatively short. The same goes for off-shoots of emo. We are about to delve into a subgenre of heavy metal, called metalcore, which was synonymous with emo by the mid 00's, so a quick low-down of the subgenre is in order. Metalcore is a linear genre of easy-to-learn song formats and structures. The key to metalcore is heavy guitar riffing in the verses, designed to show off some face-melting virtuoso play; followed by catchy choruses that listeners can sing along to; and a crescendo of the breakdown, which is a stripped and "broken down" part of the song featuring synchronized rhythm and melody timing patterns with little to no melodic differences between instruments. During the breakdown, the vocalist screams their most memorable taglines, encouraging the crowd to join and follow the danceable 4/4 lead in a moshpit.

Genre differentiation aside, metalcore joined forces with many other subgenres of punk and metal to fortify the emo scene. These subgenres became one with the emo scene by addressing the same lyrical content as standard emos.

Underoath was a metalcore band hailing from Tampa, Florida that formed in 1999. They began as a vehemently Christian band, and eventually shook off the title of a Christian band in recent years, around 2018. Whatever their religion, their albums, since day one, have addressed mental health. Their earliest work, An Act of Depression, tackled issues related to depression, suicide, and sexual abuse. After a major lineup, business model, and sound overhaul, the band became poster boy emos, and their music still reflected the same issues. On the album, They're Only Chasing Safety, "I Don't Feel Very Receptive Today," features a depressed narrator describing his experience and mentions self-mutilation "I feel like cutting it open tonight, tonight / And falling on the floor." This exact type of self-harm, namely cutting oneself, became what seemed to be an epidemic within the emo culture, but there will be more to say of the self-harm controversies in the next chapter.

Another significant emo influence from the metalcore community, We Came as Romans, was part of the movement to talk about mental health. Instead of just expressing mental health issues and giving them the spotlight, We Came As Romans promoted helping others through their trying times. In songs like "To Plant a Seed," they attempted to give voice to the "unsaid lines" of those whose "tongues are tied / to trying times." They saw the emo scene as a community of family taking care of each other and supporting each other throughout difficulty. We find their musical philosophy of radical compassion in lyrics such as:

> "I have never been so consumed
> And I have never loved it more
> [Than] To be devoted to letting all see
> What it is to live in the love of others;
> To live in the love of my brothers
> And spilling back all that anyone has ever spilled for me;
> To show that to those who have never seen."

Bands were aware of their influence on the troubled youth and began taking a step towards supporting their fans through trying times. The scene became a beacon of hope to many young people, which was part of the reason why it flooded the media and exploded in the tabloids.

However, now that emo was on the world stage, the world was watching, and the world was stunned. Upon first glance, the general population was appalled, mortified, enraged, and hostile. Of course, not everyone cared about emo, and many had ranging and mixed reviews. However, the emo scene fell prey to vicious attacks in the mainstream media. Its eccentric and outstanding fashion caught people's eyes. The intensely emotional (and often aggressive and noisy) music created an easy target for media outlets and internet bloggers to fire away. They unleashed the cannons of shaming, devaluing, rejecting, laughing, and, most importantly, blaming. As we will see, the emo scene became a source of blame for youth corruption, specifically causing teen suicide and self-harm.

After all the hard work the scene had done to create a space to talk about mental illness and help those who struggle, others accused it of creating the issues they tried to address seriously.

Media's Response (Not Huge Fans)

Recommended Listens:

1. Suicide Solution - Ozzy Osbourne
2. Better by You, Better Than Me - Judas Priest
3. Mother - Danzig
4. Shelter Me - Cinderella
5. Irresponsible Hate Anthem - Marilyn Manson
6. Du hast - Rammstein
7. Search & Destroy - KMFDM
8. Wormboy - Marilyn Manson
9. Ironic - Alanis Morissette

Blame is a funny thing. Asking "why" something is happening, finding a reason or a cause is something people always feel the need to do. Everyone has an opinion. There seems to be a constant competition to see who can say theirs louder — who can convince more people, especially on mainstream media and the internet. News channels compete to get more viewers, Youtubers compete to get more subscribers, Influencers compete to get more followers.

Alternative music has been the target for placing blame on violent events for ages. Over time, getting worse as the internet and media sources become more widely used and popularized. No matter where you look for information on the "emo" scene, you'll find someone with an opinion about what it is, where it came from, and why people are attracted to it. Media lays the blame for violence and tragedy on pop culture entertainment, often contradicting itself with misconceptions and misinformation. In turn, artists and writers blame the press for being caustic to the same issues, usually having some truth behind their thoughts.

When the Columbine shootings happened, Marilyn Manson was blamed for the victims' actions. Lamentably enough, this extreme response of putting the blame on a music genre, artist, or scene, rather than blaming the real underlying illnesses, is a typical response to alternative music.

Music is relative. It always has been, and it always will be. An artist isn't writing a song directed at children, telling them to kill themselves or others. Often, the artist tells a story based on experience from their own lives, usually utilizing metaphors and hyperbole. Music considered second, third, and fourth wave emo serve as our contemporary examples. These stories often hold positive and anti-suicide messages behind them. This positivity isn't what Fox News will tell you, though. When you Google "fox news emo," you don't find interviews with musicians or researched education pieces. Instead, you find propagandic broadcasts meant as PSA warnings for parents (and many responses to them).

Starting around the 1980s, music criticism strayed away from technical analysis and personal taste towards more sinister and severe allegations. The claim that alternative music, especially rock (heavy metal, punk, eventually emo) music can, and will cause teen suicide, gained popularity and generated waves of moral panic between 1980 to 2015.

In 1985, shock-rocker Ozzy Osbourne and his label CBS Records were brought to court on the charge that the song "Suicide Solution" from Blizzard of Oz (1981) had caused 19-year-old John McCullom to commit suicide. The case lasted well over a year before being dismissed because the First Amendment protects song lyrics. The parents of McCullom made many allegations, like believing the song contained hidden messages suggesting the listener commit suicide. Or that Ozzy and the parties in collaboration to produce the song were irresponsible for releasing it "with the knowledge that such [a song] would, or at the very least, could promote suicide."

Osbourne defended his song, explaining that "Suicide Solution" was written about the death of AC/DC's Bon Scott. Therefore, it carried a socially positive "anti-suicide" message. Bob Daisley — bassist and lyricist for several solo Ozzy records, wrote this "Suicide Solution" alongside Ozzy. Although Ozzy was thinking of Bon Scott's death when writing, Daisley had Ozzy's excessive drug and alcohol tendencies in mind. However you look at it, when considering the genuine thoughts behind the song, the meaning is anti-suicide.

Similarly, in 1990, Judas Priest and CBS Records were brought to court to face charges against them concerning a double-suicide pact. The song "Better By You, Better Than Me" from Stained Class (1978) allegedly caused the suicide of Raymond Belnap and the attempted suicide of his friend James Vance. After Vance recovered, he and his parents sued the band for supposedly having hidden subliminal messages like "try suicide," "do it," and "let's be dead" in the song. It was a bogus case, lasting a straight month, causing lasting distress to both the band and the grieving parents. The court exonerated the band.

Rob Hafford, lead singer of Judas Priest, in a Rolling Stone article, remembers thinking, "Why are we here? We're British metal musicians, and we're having to defend ourselves and our music and our fans about the ridiculous, absurd accusations that we put these messages in our music designed to kill yourself. It was preposterous, absolutely ridiculous. So it was a very emotional circumstance... I really wanted to go over to the mother of the boy who killed himself and give her a hug, and say, 'I'm sorry for the loss of your kid. Let's go have a coffee and talk this over.'" He acknowledges that the parents were angry — and rightfully so, but the anger was pointed in the wrong direction.
Tipper Gore, co-founder of the Parents Music Resource Center (PMRC), fed into this disdain for rock music for years. In 1987, she

published a book called Raising PG Kids in an X-Rated Society. She suggested that further than censorship and rating albums, rock music "should be stopped — not labeled, debated, or criticized."

Contents	
Introduction	11
1. A Mother Takes a Stand	15
2. Where Have All the Children Gone?	39
3. The Cult of Violence	47
4. Selling More Than the Sizzle: Explicit Sex in the Media	81
5. Merchants of Death: Touting Teen Suicide	103
6. Playing with Fire: Heavy Metal Satanism	117
7. The Medium Is the Mixer: Alcohol and Drugs in Entertainment	127
8. Rockin' and Shockin' in the Concert Free-for-All Zone	143
9. Parenting in an Explicit Society	157
Conclusion	165
Appendix A	169
Appendix B	175
Notes	193
Index	209

Knowing that an extinction of rock wouldn't happen, she led the PMRC to take multiple types of action against rock music. They had a heavy hand in pressuring label companies to tag albums with warnings that read "Parental Advisory: Explicit Lyrics," and rating music in terms of X-rated (sexually explicit), or R-rated (containing violence, profanity, occult, glorification of drugs & alcohol).

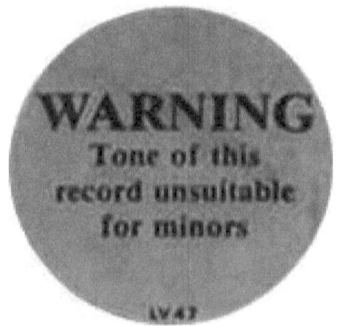

(early version used in the 1980s)

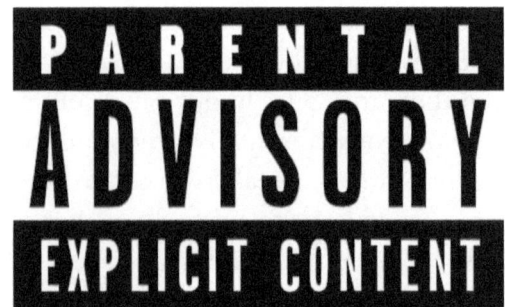

(current label, introduced in 1996)

Musicians reacted to Tipper Gore and the **PMRC** by calling them out and ridiculing them in their songs and on stage during live shows. Danzig's song "Mother" (1988) is a direct protest to the censorship mindset, singing,

>Mother [Tipper Gore]
>Tell your children not to walk my way
>Tell your children not to hear my words [Advisory label]
>What they mean
>{claim that artists were harming children}
>What they say
>Mother
>Mother
>Can you keep them in the dark for life?
>{rhetorical questions}
>Can you hide them from the waiting world?
>Oh mother

Cinderella also expresses their indignation of Gore in their song, "Shelter Me" (1990) by singing,

>Tipper led the war against the record industry
>She said she saw the devil on her MTV

This is a song that ultimately opposes the claim that music is causing harm, and rather argues that it is a coping mechanism for hard times. Keifer sings,

>Everybody needs a little place they can hide
>Somewhere to call their own
>Don't let nobody inside
>Every now and then we all need to let go
>For some it's a doctor, for me it's rock and roll

One of the many negative consequences that came from these accusations and allegations was a myth that is still often believed in, even though it has been debunked by psychologists and correlating research and studies. It is called the "Copycat," "Werther," or "cluster effect" syndrome. It became a popular myth regarding teen suicide, and has still been used incorrectly by mainstream media outlets. The "copycat" syndrome — in that teens are thought to imitate the suicides of others (whether celebrities, friends, or anonymous victims). For example, when Kurt Cobain of Nirvana was tragically found dead from suicide, a wave of rumours began shortly after - claiming that teen suicides saw an immediate spike and were believed to be connected to Cobain's suicide.

Approximately 90 out of 100 kids who commit suicide meet a psychiatric diagnosis. Kids are not just killing themselves just because they've been treated harshly or life's seemingly dealt them a bad hand. There is an internal process going on. Organizations like the American Association of Suicidology can help provide information for those who may be at risk. It is not always clear when people are communicating thoughts of suicide, so it is essential to pay attention to warning signs.

More subtle warning signs may include (increased) substance abuse, behavioural changes like severe withdrawal or apathy, frequent depressive episodes involving a change in sleep patterns, or loss of appetite. More serious warning signs may be individuals making final arrangements like giving away belongings or finding long term care for their animals.

Now that we've outlined some of the outrageous claims that initiated the war between music and censorship, we can move into the waves of moral panic that followed. We argue that there were two peak waves of moral panic.

The first wave being from 1996 to 1999 and revolving around Marilyn Manson. Manson created his stage persona in 1989 to "be the loudest, most persistent alarm clock [he] could be because there didn't seem like any other way to snap society out of its Christianity and media-induced coma." He made it his mission to shock America through topics of death, disease, violence, betrayal, disillusionment, and more, in an attempt to "liberate" people. In his second studio album, Antichrist Superstar, released in 1996, he socially critiques modern culture. Manson describes US conservatism's fascist elements, the censorship war, and mocks the claims that rock music causes teen suicide.

In the opening track, "Irresponsible Hate Anthem," it opens with "I am so all-American / I'd sell you suicide." In "Mr. Superstar," he maintains the theme with, "Hey Mr. Superstar / I'd kill myself for you." He goes against the "copycat" myth that young people kill themselves because they've been influenced by celebrities committing suicide. The song "Tourniquet" compares an emergency tool that stops blood loss in limb injuries to media making Manson the poster boy for objectionable motifs and cause of violent events. In the single's chorus, he wails, "Take your hatred out on me / Make your victim my head / You never ever believed in me / I am your tourniquet."

Similarly, in "Wormboy," a rough voice tells the story of a protagonist worm who "gets his wings," which grants them power and popularity of society's elite but wanting to rebel against them. Two voices repeatedly take turns — a high pitch voice screeching, "Oh no, I am," and a gritty voice following it up with, "All the things they said I was." This story parallels Manson's life as he was becoming a pop culture icon. As the Canadian pop legacy, Alanis Morissette, would say, "and isn't it ironic."

Disturbingly enough, following the release of this "social critique" album, the mainstream media obsession with Manson spiked when a 15-year-old boy, Richard Kuntz, committed suicide. His father blamed it on Marilyn Manson and the Antichrist Superstar album. This claim prompted a US Senate Subcommittee hearing on "Music Violence: How Does it Affect Our Youth?" This hearing disgracefully dragged Kuntz' death through the mud, while mainly targeting Manson.

In Senator Lieberman's opening statement to the hearing, he (inaccurately) compares Manson's music to that of Cannibal Corpse — a band who capitalizes, if not glorifies, topics like abuse, suicide, and murder to intentionally disturb listeners. He makes his beliefs on music culture and Manson known, calling them "vile, hateful, nihilistic, and, as you will hear from Mr. Kuntz, dangerously damaging music." Mr. Kuntz does, in fact, hold these same beliefs. In a letter addressing Lieberman asking to speak at this hearing, he claimed, "the music wasn't symptomatic of other problems. I would say that the music caused him to kill himself."

He followed up with, "I failed to recognize that my son was holding a hand grenade [the Antichrist Superstar CD] and it was live and that it was going to go off in his mind." To which Lieberman replied, "don't be too hard on yourself … it didn't look like a hand grenade. It looked like a CD." Following this hearing, throughout 1997 and 1998, talk shows and news programs were inundated with devastated and grievous parents desperately claiming linkages between Manson's music and their child's self-inflicted deaths.

In April of 1999, one of the most culture-rocking tragedies occurred, spinning America into a media feeding frenzy. In Littleton, Colorado, at Columbine High School, 12 students and one teacher were shot dead by teenagers Eric Harris and Dylan Klebold, who later killed themselves. This shooting was publicized in detail, with multitudes of speculation and falsely laying blame. During the dawn of modern technology, the internet was becoming more widely used. Many new outlets demonized their hobbies and scrutinized bands like Marilyn Manson, trying to find something to blame for these shootings.

Media allowed floods of content on the shooters and how they planned their atrocity to become widely accessible. The boys planned the shooting meticulously, including leaving behind manifesto's and video journals to be found so that their story might outlive them. Unfortunately, it did. This tragic event was not the first but was arguably the most influential shooting — inspiring (among many other reasons), for instance, 20-year-old Adam Lanza to shoot down 20 children and six staff at Sandy Hook Elementary in Newton, Connecticut.

With no apparent reason why they would commit such an act, the media blamed their fashion choices and music taste. Ultimately condemning a form of entertainment for causing the shooting. False claims from student witnesses remark that the boys were a part of a group called the "Trench Coat Mafia," and they were fans of Marilyn Manson. The claims were formally rescinded from the official investigation. However, mainstream media and public speculation refused to let go of these claims, blaming Manson for the event for years following.

The level of infamy Manson reached for the blame of Columbine was unforeseeable, even to him. Initially, he refused "to jump into the media frenzy" and defend himself, even after discovering that the boys weren't fans of his music. In late May 1999, with insufferable public pressure and insistence from his label, Manson went on record in an open letter to the Columbine killings through Rolling Stone. In this letter, he reiterates the critique of American society that has been so forcefully articulated in his music:

> "When it comes down to who's to blame for the high school murders in Littleton, Colorado, throw a rock and you'll hit someone who's guilty. We're the people who sit back and tolerate children owning guns, and we're the ones who tune in and watch the up-to-the-minute details of what they do with them. I think it's terrible when anyone dies, especially if it is someone you know and love...I was dumbfounded as I watched the media snake right in, not missing a teardrop, interviewing the parents of dead children, televising the funerals. Then came the witch hunt."

Later, he flips the question around:

> "Even if they were fans, that gives them no excuse, nor does it mean that music is to blame. Did we look for James Huberty's inspiration when he gunned down people at McDonald's? What did Timothy McVeigh like to watch? What about David Koresh, Jim Jones? Do you think entertainment inspired Kip Kinkel, or should we blame the fact that his father bought him the guns he used in the Springfield, Oregon, murders? What inspires Bill Clinton to blow people up in Kosovo? Was it something that Monica Lewinsky said to him? Isn't killing just killing, regardless if it's in Vietnam or Jonesboro, Arkansas? Why do we justify one, just because it seems to be for the right reasons? Should there ever be a right reason?"

A few years later, Manson was interviewed in Michael Moore's 2002 Bowling for Columbine documentary. The band was involved in legal action against those who used their name, explicitly blaming their music for the shooting. Manson has said in multiple interviews that the allegations nearly took everything from him and destroyed his career. In this interview with Moore, he says, "I can see why they would pick me. It's easy to throw my face on the screen. I'm a poster boy for fear, because I represent what they're afraid of, because I do and say what I want … It's a campaign of fear and consumption."

And when asked if he could say something to the kids at Columbine school, what would he say — he responded, "I wouldn't say a single word to them. I would listen, 'cuz that's what no one did."

The tragedy that was the Columbine school shooting, and the many others that have followed it, pushed conversations away from what was causing teen suicide. Instead, it focused more on gun violence, gun control, carrying rights, and public safety protocols. This waned the panic revolving around allegations made against alternative music until 2006 — when the second wave of moral panic crashed, engulfing mainstream media in questions and accusations surrounding "emo" culture. From 2006 to 2008, mainstream media and the general public fed into a negative stigmatism of "emo" culture, helping create divides between genre fans and between parents and their children.

... Moral Panic (Pt. II)

Recommended Listens:

1. I Will Follow You into the Dark - Death Cab for Cutie
2. Famous Last Words - My Chemical Romance
3. We Are The Others - Delain

"Emo Undercover: Report on Emo/Scene Kids" was a Fox News broadcast aired in 2006. It began a mainstream thought that "emo" was a sudden internet sensation that exploded out of thin air, which lured kids into its sadistic and evil subculture. The report starts off telling parents what emo's look like: it's a fashion statement after all. Androgynous looks via tight girl jeans, makeup, and multicoloured hair. The video goes on a lengthy explanation of the "emo" scene, where they narrow in on rare extremes, twisting the perception of the scene to a surface level where kids idolize confessionals and self-mutilation for reasons no deeper than being influenced by entertainment and emo culture.

The report displays inter-scene genre divides, where goths, heavy metalheads, and punk-rocker [older generational] types infamously ridiculed and tormented emo's. A Youtube video surfaced for "The Emo Song" by Adam and Andrew — a group that primarily releases parody and ridicule songs with transphobic, homophobic, hyper-masculine themes, and stigmatizes mental illness and self-harm — which are the precise themes and messages in the song. A "Beatdown Day" was hosted on 06-06-06 to target anyone tormentors could find who looked like an "emo," and beat them relentlessly while filming it so other bullies could share in the ridicule online. This targeting of emo's, goths, and anyone who looked different or expressed themselves in this type of style, became a hate crime that was seen in the community all too often, and for a long time, with no real consequences.

The broadcast showed clips displaying even more antipathy, like "Emocide," an anti-emo festival held by death metal fans. There was a two-part YouTube video called "Emo Assault Squadron," where Zachary Byron Helm and "the Agents of SORP" act as police officers who hunt down emos and "curb stomp" them, using derogatory and aggressively stigmatic terms through the whole narrative. Helm was shown in this news report saying, "Emo is kind of like a pansy version of the Goths, so in a way, it's almost our duty to give them a little bit of crap."

The report focused on divisions in the community, negative perceptions, and misinformation. Doing so pushed aside the real reasons behind children who self-harmed and had suicidal thoughts or tendencies, who were experiencing depression, anxiety, and more. It also interfered in getting them help by creating fear and panic in parents instead of suggesting an open dialogue based on a child's psychological or behavioural red flags.

In 2007, ABC News broadcasted a report they introduced as "Emo: PSA." It was "a warning to parents about a trend that is causing self-mutilation and suicide … in a state where teen suicide is at an all-time high — every parent should know about the so-called 'emo' culture." This broadcast reiterates the myth that emo "came out of the internet and into the lives of teens." This report again focuses on extremes and heavily feeds into the negative stigmatism of the perception of "emo."

They describe the average "emo" as filled with "sadness, rage, and pain in the form of self-harm," while showing parody and fad sites like an "emo quiz." In this special, they interview a 15-year-old boy, Ritch Tanner, who had scars and cuts on his wrists from self-harm and was not shy about showing them off. This boy was unhealthy — his father reported him missing and described him as "ill, and displaying some traits of 'emo' culture that are disturbing to psychologists and parents." The boy had an ongoing history and battle with mental illness, and this report brushed over the seriousness of this, and instead painted Ritch Tanner as just another average "emo."

At one point in the report, they tell parents that "suicide is the #2 cause of deaths among teens and link suicide to 'emo' culture." Following up with an example of this so-called toxic suicidal culture, they play a clip of "I Will Follow You Into the Dark" by Death Cab for Cutie. In reality, as Ben Gibbard told in an interview about the song, it was written in 15 or 20 minutes after the phrase, "I will follow you into the dark," passed through his mind on the cab to the studio. It "was beamed down to him" after weeks of struggling to write in the studio. Gibbard connects the theme to the fact that eventually, everyone dies, including ourselves. The main idea was mortality, not suicide. Death is an ever-impending reality. "Writing a love song that talks about the inevitable death of one's partner, and that you will eventually follow that person into whatever the afterlife is or is not, is something people can relate to." Mortality is what's at the heart of the song.

The 2007 news report also depicts images on "gender-bending," which they explain in a homophobic way — by showing photos of gay couples kissing and repeating that because boys are often wearing girls' pants and makeup, they are "exploring the [gender] boundaries."

They almost start to head in a better direction when they feature a psychologist on the screen informing parents not to approach the topic with fear, that not all kids that look like a part of "emo" culture cut themselves — but if any parent does find evidence of cutting, they should put their child into therapy: "[the] key is to understand the deeper reasons why their child draws to 'emo' culture in the first place." The report itself contradicts that conclusion by showing extremes of the culture, biasedly giving parents "signs to look out for" like the fashion statement, rather than asking more questions to understand children's struggles. This moral panic wave climaxed in 2008 when The Daily Mail ran yet another slam piece calling emo a "suicide cult." Titled, "Why No Child is Safe from This Sinister Cult of Emo," the article focused on 13-year-old Hannah Bond, who took her own life "just three months after becoming an emo." The article made national news by revealing that Hannah was "obsessed" with My Chemical Romance (MCR). The coroner, Roger Sykes, stated that Hannah took her own life because "she was thinking about how this [suicide] would go down with those others who were involved with the emo fad." The article held factual inaccuracies, such as declaring that "Black Parade was a place where all emos believe they go when they die," as if MCR's third album was some twisted, pseudo-religious propaganda.

The report was so contradictory to what MCR and music fans truly believed that a protest outside of The Daily Mail occurred, where over 300 protestors held signs that read, "MCR saves lives," "I'm not afraid to keep on living," (a lyric from "Famous Last Words" on The Black Parade album), and "We're not a Cult — we're an Army!" Parents of teenaged MCR fans organized the protest. No one said it better than one mother and fan of MCR, Caz Hill, who explained the protestor's point of view; which included her teenage daughters, saying, "I was furious with the Daily Mail for falsely reporting that My Chemical Romance promoted suicide and their fans were a cult. It cashed in on parents' fears of the emo culture. The Daily Mail took a young girl's tragic death and outrageously claimed she took her own life after listening to My Chemical Romance, which made her want to "join the Black Parade." How sick and irresponsible can a publication be?" (our emphasis).

Unfortunately, like many other social issues, someone had to die before we started seeing meaningful consequences. On August 11, 2007, in Bacup, Lancashire, England, 20-year-old Sophie Lancaster and her partner, Rob Maltby, were "set upon in a vicious and completely unprovoked attack by a large group of teenagers." Both were repeatedly kicked in the head and left bleeding and unconscious. Rob eventually emerged from his coma but Sophie never did. She passed away on August 24, 2007.

The attackers shouted something like, "Let's bang the moshers!" This couple was attacked solely because they looked and expressed themselves through fashion differently than others. In a small town, Sophie was instantly recognizable with her multiple facial piercings and often multicoloured dreadlocks. She was a vegetarian, an advocate for identifying issues like world poverty, and was a voracious reader. Sophie's mother, Sylvia, described the couple as "bright, creative, intelligent people."

Following the attack, Silvia launched the SOPHIE campaign, standing for Stamp Out Prejudice, Hatred, and Intolerance Everywhere. At the time, she still expected Sophie to make a full recovery. Once Sophie died, the campaign gained momentum as bands, celebrities, alternative communities, online groups, and ordinary people embraced the message of tolerance and acceptance. This campaign turned into the Sophie Lancaster Foundation. It focuses on "creating respect for the understanding of subcultures in our communities." It became a registered charity in 2009 and works in conjunction with politicians and police forces to ensure the law protects individuals who are part of subcultures. In 2013, Greater Manchester Police became the first to monitor and record hate crimes and incidents against people from Alternative Subcultures, with several other police authorities following by example. In 2014, Sylvia was awarded a "Most Excellent Order of the British Empire" (OBE) for "Community Cohesion — Especially in Reduction of Hate Crime." The foundation still has an active website.

Children have always been looking to fit in, find themselves, and figure out why they were put on this planet. Growing up is a chaotic whirlwind, filled with half-developed ideas and flying by the seat of your pants. What happens when you're a kid that can't seem to fit into any group of friends, can't relate to the plethora of pop culture TV shows playing on your older siblings screen, who doesn't feel like your parents listen to or understand you? Well, you search desperately for someone, something, to ease the loneliness and confusion.

For kids who found the "emo" scene, it was often a turning point for the better. With just a few clicks, especially in the early-present 2000s, you can find music that screams what you're feeling, friends on sites who feel the same disconnect to their surroundings, and comfort in knowing you're not the only one feeling out of the ordinary — you're not alone. And so, what happens when the community and solace you've found comes under attack? Well, you defend it.

PART THREE:
OUT OF THE MOSHPIT, INTO THE CLINIC, THEN BACK TO THE MOSHPIT

Did Music Save My Life?

Recommended Listens:

1. Ohio Is for Lovers - Hawthorne Heights
2. Headfirst for Halos - My Chemical Romance
3. Faith in the Knife - Scary Kids Scaring Kids
4. People You Know - Dance Gavin Dance
5. Wanderlust - Every Time I Die
6. People Who Died - Against Me!; from Songs That Saved My Life
7. Real World - State Champs; from Songs That Saved My Life Vol.2

While it is indisputable that the various waves of emo did a great deal to further mental health discourse within mainstream culture, the positive net effect of some of these individual contributions is dubious. Not all messages about or related to mental health are helpful, and some may push listeners further away from dealing with their ailments properly.

The elephant in the room, particularly regarding third wave emo, is undoubtedly the genre's association with self-harm. As far as the greater culture was concerned, emo and "slitting wrists" were synonymous. This perception was cemented in 2008, when the parents of a British teenager who committed suicide blamed emo culture for her death. Media outlets parroted the story, thus they permanently instilled the idea that self-harm was a rite of passage for emos.

There is some academic literature that may provide support for the assertion that emo promotes cutting in teens. A study of 4,000 teens found that people belonged to alternative subcultures (emo, punks, and metal fans) were three times more likely to self-harm as well as a six times higher risk of suicide, as well as experience victimization and hate crimes. So much so, the researchers suggested the advent of specialist support services with strategies geared to helping the said demographic.

In some cases, it may be that people prone to depression and subsequent symptoms are naturally attracted to these subcultures, as opposed to the underground scenes inciting such conditions. That said, even after adjusting their study for factors such as previous depression, victimization, and histories of self-harm, the study found that contact with alternative subcultures still increased their predisposition to these behaviours.

Later on, two qualitative papers would come out supporting assertions that self-harm and suicide were normalized via subcultures like emo and detailed possible mechanisms that enabled this to happen. Ultimately, a review of the papers found there is currently limited support for the proposed mechanisms. The lead researcher would go on to say "there is currently not adequate evidence to draw conclusions that these alternative subcultures themselves are in any way harmful." Still, the studies do substantiate some self-reflection on the way mental health issues were portrayed in third wave emo.

Certainly, there are many lyrics in third wave emo that could at least be interpreted to praise behaviour like self-harm. For example, the Hawthorne Heights song, "Ohio is for Lovers," contains the sing-along refrain, "So cut my wrists and black my eyes / So I can fall asleep tonight, or die." In fairness, the lyrics are taken out of context and are but a single piece of a greater metaphor that is not meant to promote self-harm, but this nuance could be lost on an impressionable and young fan base. Similarly, in the My Chemical Romance song, "Headfirst for Halos," lead singer Gerard Way seethes, "And I think I'll blow my brains against the ceiling / and as the fragments of my skull begin to fall / fall on your tongue like pixie dust / just think happy thoughts we'll fly home."

In response to accusations of being an "emo suicide cult," My Chemical Romance issued a statement clarifying, "our lyrics are about finding the strength to keep living through pain and hard times." Perhaps this sentiment had been lost on some members of their fan base in a wash of grim visuals and catch-phrase lines that proved to be more salient than the wholesome meaning underpinning it all. Emo had carved out a niche for itself by embracing such pronounced melodramaticism. It raises several questions: Do artists have a responsibility to consider the message retention of their young and impressionable audiences? Do these sorts of lyrics run the risk of commodifying real mental health issues into some sort of tribal symbol?

Even more, the darker (albeit, much rarer and less mainstream) underbelly of third wave emo contained some messages that were pitch black without any underlying redemptive qualities. The song, "Faith in the Knife," by Scary Kids Scaring Kids contains lyrics, "Find me some beauty in this deceptive place / Before you know it, I'll be gone without a trace," and, "Nothing this good could last forever / I put all my faith in this knife / The lust feels like the tears fall from your eyes." Here, there is no greater metaphor, or spin on the lyrics that urges the listener to keep on. Quite the opposite, it is bleak and paints no way out. While there may be an argument that some may have felt relief in knowing they were not alone in having such dark thoughts, one could easily imagine a 12 or 13-year old fan receiving questionable values and suggestions from this track.

Now, to be fair to third-wave emo, the situation was not black and white. A wide variety of demographics comprised the emo scene. With the diverse demographics came diverse economic and social situations that played a role in determining how the entire scene, bands and fans included, responded to their overt relationship to mental illness.

To begin with, major bands in the third-wave scene challenged stigmas surrounding the scene by metafictionally addressing the irresponsible ways that bands promote their mental health problems. For example, in the Dance Gavin Dance song, "People You Know" the narrator wishes to write a song that connects to his audience, screaming: "Someone please! / Please write a script that's made for me / That appeals to people listening to this CD." The narrator then describes what that script would look like and portrays a typical scene vocalist connecting to his audience at a show: "Rancid is the sound of my voice / Croaking its drama across an orchestra of friendly faces / Singing along with their dying concern." However, the vocalist is a self-deprecating narcissist who uses their privilege for selfish ends.

> I am a prick, look at me go
> I can get lucky playing some shows, I'm a bitch
> I'ma go get some new expensive shit
> Oh man I hurt
> Emotions they suck
> But I'll just tell people,
> "I don't give a fuck about that shit."

The vocalist clearly knows he feels inner turmoil and pain but neglects, refusing professional help in favor of self-medication — "I need money / I need clothes / I need women / I need blow." Though it seems that the song is endorsing such a selfish pattern of deflection, immediately after this line, a musical break occurs. The narrator interjects ironically, "something is very fucking wrong." The narrator concludes that the script made for him is morally corrupt, and he explicitly announces that fact amongst what seems to be his real personal story.

Another interesting example of third-wave artists using irony to denounce the scene's messy treatment of mental health is the band Everytime I Die. They are a hardcore band that reached a high point in the scene during the third wave. Due to the aggressive, angry, and male-dominated nature of hardcore music, Everytime I Die had to maintain the stereotypical appearance of a violently masculine rage band. In an interview regarding their album The New Junk Aesthetic, singer Keith Buckley explained "the junk aesthetic pertains to the fact that there is a lot of shitty art out there, and you don't know what is art and what is garbage." We can say the same applied to artists' treatment of mental health in the scene — many fans didn't know what was art and what was garbage.

So, to go beyond the hardcore stereotype, the band simultaneously embraced and denied it. The New Junk Aesthetic sounds gritty, raw, brutal, and unrelenting. The unnamed main character confidently (or so it seems) struts self-hatred, gluttony, depression, and abuse. Amidst the chaos, the narrator announces at the end of "Wanderlust," "When they unearth these passages / Will I appear to be proud? / Not if you're listening close enough / Not if you're sounding it out." Everytime I Die had to work around their tough-guy image to give their audience the music they desired while also expressing their desire to address mental health.

To further complicate third-wave's relationship with mental health, though there is not reliable academic literature, we can say anecdotally that a large portion of people in the emo scene were not in privileged positions. Each individual has a different story, but generally the emo age groups were younger, so they did not know how to access mental health resources properly. Further, they likely could not afford treatments and medication in privatized health care systems. Additionally, there were multiple other factors, including stigma around treatment, familial and peer acceptance of treatment, and geographical access to mental health resources.

In the 1990s, psychology experienced the decade of the brain, where researchers introduced many of the psychiatric medications used today. These medications, along with proper therapy, were not available or wholly developed all across America (and still aren't in many places). So, although there were often massive faults or controversial takes regarding mental health within the emo scene's depictions and treatment of it, the scene was making the best of what it was given. Further, given the young demographic of the scene, they could hardly be expected to know the academic literature regarding mental health nor could they be trusted to find out about it without assistance. The emo scene, moreover, began to see that they lacked the resources, so they began to use their obviously influential platform to strive for better education and access to mental health resources.

Fourth Wave: Defending Pop-Punk: Sliding Into the 2010s on a Pizza Skateboard

Recommended Listens:

1. The Great Repetition - Touché Amoré
2. Mental Health - The World Is A Beautiful Place & I Am No Longer Afraid To Die
3. (*trigger warning!*) In Framing - The Hotelier
4. Your Deep Rest - The Hotelier
5. Re-done - Modern Baseball
6. The Stigma (Boys Don't Cry) - AS IT IS
7. The End. - AS IT IS
8. Don't Let Me Cave In - The Wonder Years
9. The Devil In My Bloodstream - The Wonder Years
10. Cardinals - The Wonder Years
11. From The Outside - Real Friends
12. Smiling On The Surface - Real Friends
13. Untitled - Knuckle Puck
14. Overexposed - Sleep On It

Emo's meteoric rise in mainstream culture began to cool off towards the end of the aughts. Staples of emo fashion were subsequently borrowed by other subculture movements (such as hipsters, eboys and egirls, and ravers) and the mainstream, once again returning emo to relative ambiguity. Still, the mainstream popularity had enshrined emo as one of the more popular underground music scenes for years to come. Vans Warped Tour, for example, persisted into the late 2010s, featuring emo artists in the largest travelling festival in the United States. These emo bands, primarily pop-punk and metalcore acts, began to shift the discourse of emo once again.

Whereas the emos of the aughts primarily discussed teenage relationships woes and feelings of despair, the 2010 bands began to shine a light on feelings of anxiety and lacking direction. Whereas emos of the aughts had embraced a sleek layer of pop-radio production on their music, fourth wave emo bands embraced rawer, more abrasive mixes — a concession to the anticommercialism of the first and second wave emo's. These acts were the catalyst for a brief resurgence of emo music in 2012 (although they ultimately achieved only a fraction the popularity of mid-aughts emo acts), which tended to focus on an older, college-aged demographic.

So what is the fourth wave of emo? Well it started from two concurrent streams, which were never disconnected but remained distinct: Defend Pop-Punk and emo revival.

Emo revival wanted to bring the 1st and 2nd wave emo sounds back to life, sounds which the 3rd wave mainstream pop-esque sound had drowned out. The emo revival scene moved back to the raw mixing, hardcore influence, and loosey-goosey song structure, formatting, and standards. Major emo revival bands include Citizen, Title Fight, Touché Amoré, Turnover, The Front Bottoms, Spanish Love Songs, Into it. Over it., Balance and Composure, and The World is a Beautiful Place and I am No Longer Afraid To Die.

These emo revival bands wanted to reconnect with mental health in a more honest way than they may have perceived third wave emo's response to mental health issues. Disregarding form and standards was not just an aesthetic move that sounded cool to them, but the messy, aggressive, and sloppy sounds of emo revival gave a sincere take to the ugliness, pain, and chaos of mental illnesses, particularly depression and anxiety.

For example, on the song "The Great Repetition," by Touche Amore, melancholy chords compliment an aggressive, hardcore sounding mix, as the vocalist screams a comparison between his suicidal thoughts and a dramatic performance:

> "This is my final act
> So I'll need your full attention
> And for my final trick
> I'll make everyone who loves me disappear
> But I won't know
> How to bring them back."

Emo revival bands did not want to dilute their emotion or cloud the feeling of mental illness with catchy riffs and radio-playable choruses, and bands like Touche Amore made an effort to take over the underground scene while staying true to their messages.

Emo revival bands didn't just want to confess their mental health issues like the 1st and 2nd wave did, struggling to find audiences willing to acceptingly listen to their confessionals. At this point, the door to mental health conversations had swung wide open. Emo revival bands wanted to use that open door to, as best as possible, communicate about mental health truthfully. This desire to truthfully communicate did not make its fulfillment easy. In fact the songwriter's difficulty ramped up in some aspects when artists set a goal of accurately representing their emotions because such accuracy is a tall order. Hence, bands went back to using sonic qualities and more subtle lyrical metaphors to explain themselves.

Another example of an emo revival band using their throwback sound to reconnect with their emotional roots is The World is a Beautiful Place and I am No Longer Afraid to Die. Indeed, their name alone is worth thinking about because it suggests a powerful story. The "I" is stating that the world is something valuable and good and the crippling fear he had about death has dissipated, likely because "I" sees the world in a new and wondrous light. The song "Mental Health" by The World is a Beautiful Place relays some feelings and asks questions that people with mental illness dwell on like "Do you remember the start / where it all came down?" The narrator also reminds their addressee that it's "Better to let them know / Sooner than later," that is, it's better to open up to friends and family who can help you get the attention you need. The narrator also consoles their friend, confidently stating "you are normal and healthy to forgive yourself" for their limitations.

As a final example, The Hotelier's album, Home, Like Noplace Is There, tackles mental health as its central theme. The Hotelier combatted the toxic culture that mainstream media accused third wave emo music of glorifying by coming to grips with the harsh realities of mental health and the dark consequences of its mismanagement.

The song "In Framing" attends to the first-hand trauma of watching depression, addiction, self-harm, and suicide unfold. The song lays it on the table with gruesome details as the narrator recounts (trigger warning):

> "As you climbed out the window, your face cold as stone
> You lifted the towel, your wrist showed the bone
> I held my breath in the ER, I swayed as I stood
> I tried to stay steady to protect you the best that I could
> You pretended to sleep the entire ride home
> But I heard you crying when you felt alone."

The Hotelier refuses to romanticize the ugly and brings explicit attention to the dark side of mental illness. There are brave, courageous, and proud moments when triumphing against mental illness, but there are also lows of grief, shame, anger, and irreversible loss that we must admit openly and truthfully.

Indeed, some people never escape their illness, and sometimes it ends in tragedy. The next track on the album, "Your Deep Rest," comes to grips with grief and guilt surrounding suicide. The title is an oronym with the words "you're depressed" because the two phrases sound the same. Here, perhaps as a continuation of the previous track, the narrator feels guilty of ignoring his friend's depression, which resulted in suicide, and is too ashamed to attend the funeral. The "deep rest" of the title refers to his friend's death, and the oronymic words "you're depressed" are the words that the narrator wishes he had uttered to address his deceased friend. He bleakly sings,

> "I called in sick from your funeral
> The sight of your family made me feel responsible
> And I found the notes you left behind
> Little hints and helpless cries
> Desperate wishing to be over"

Each song on the album paints a bleak picture of unfettered, untreated, and unforgiving mental illness, which encourages listeners to face their mental health issues courageously and empathetically relate to experiences they may not know.

Defend Pop-Punk worked differently to change the movement of emo. Defend Pop-Punk was a new generation of artists and listeners who grew up listening to the third wave. What began as a surge of up and coming bands became a new era of emo unified through their ethical visions of the scene. Raised on an amalgamation of the many genres present in the third wave, fourth wave pop-punk bands embraced fans and artists alike from a wide variety of sonic backgrounds. They proposed an ethics of inclusion, empathy, and open-mindedness. They battled the stereotype of third-wave emo bands, which elevated the bands to a pedestal on which they stood as authorities, role models, and often sex symbols. They also stood out by talking honestly about their mental illness in a manner much more straightforward and explicit than ever before in the pop-punk scene.

Defend Pop-Punk was more of a mindset that began in the early emo days and was now in full bloom rather than a solitary movement organized by a group of people. However, the infamous saying "Defend Pop-Punk" originated when a band, Man Overboard, jokingly reskinned a "Defend Hardcore" shirt from an underground New York hardcore band.

Rather than a show-off bad boy mystique, Man Overboard consisted of a group of lanky, broken-hearted, and socially anxious boys who sang highschool poetry confessionals. The idea that musicians were cool, attractive, and charismatic was ingrained in even the emo culture, as their most famous stars also gathered obsessive fan bases. Man Overboard was proof that you didn't need to be conventionally handsome to sell out venues and have real love problems.

Modern Baseball was another band whose image, persona, and aura did not align with the typical fashion, expectations, and affectations of third-wave emo rockstars. Yet the band was a hit. They also changed the direction of mental health conversations within the scene. For example, they offer a more honest and factual take of social anxiety in "Re-Done," explaining:

> "I couldn't conjure words cause I thought about it too long
> So I'll leave the steady hands to Sean
> 'Cause we all know I lack
> In the field of conversing correctly
> Without shaking or getting queasy
> Not letting my emotions get involved."

The band depicts anxiety in a factual manner that is not overdramatized or exaggerated beyond belief. Their style also takes mental health seriously and attempts to express mental health issues clearly. The band unveils a realistic vision of their symptoms through traditional emo tropes, like high-school girl troubles and fitting in at parties.

Further, the band addresses the stigma that condemns the emo scene and discards their relationship with mental illness as a bunch of spoiled suburban teenage angst that will pass in time. On "Re-Done," we also hear the following ending, which stresses the need to take mental illness seriously rather than putting it at the end of a joke:

> "They just think we are young with broken hearts
> Stomping around every day
> So let's stomp around breaking
> Young at heart all the way."

They directly address the condemnation of mental illness that reduces it to people who are just "young with broken hearts." The narrator concludes that since he is misjudged by onlookers, he will no longer concern himself with them, and they will continue to mislabel him.

Though the Defend Pop-Punk movement was substantial in its own right, another considerable impact on the scene was not the artists but the fan base. After the Defend Pop-Punk rise, a dedicated group of fans emerged out of their gloomy bedroom filled to the brim with Hot Topic novelties and band merch, to form the notorious Defend Pop Punk Group. Currently sitting just shy of 31,000 members, the group is a drop spot for everything pizza, music, and emotional support. You heard me right; nothing hits the spot quite like a hot slice and a song recommendation that pulls the heartstrings harder than your junior high crush dumping you.

This group of young social justice warriors is quick to the front lines when discussing the importance of mental illness. Many of the posts on the group consist of questions like "can you give me songs to help me through my parent's divorce?" or "what are some bands that helped you through a depressive episode?" Without hesitation, group members offer support as song recommendations, but also as advice from friends in a similar situation.

For many of these younger adults and teenagers, most of the information or advice they receive is from the bands they idolize and the lyrics of their favourite songs. While this guidance is useful for sparking conversation and awareness, it can also be dangerous if misinformed. Some bands may have good intentions with their songs, but younger audiences may still easily misinterpret their messages, as we noted previously.

The lead singer of AS IT IS, Patty Walters, discussed this problem of irresponsible songwriting with Upset Magazine explaining that he did not want to be a part of this issue. Many bands in the emo scene bring comfort to individuals suffering from some form of mental illness. However, Patty claims that many of these bands "contribute to glamorizing, to romanticizing, to even fetishizing mental illness." This awareness can complicate songwriting because artists want to express their emotions, feel proud of their triumphs, and admit to the ugly parts of mental illness. Additionally, audiences want to hear music they relate to, and sometimes glamorous music sells, even when it's toxic. For Walters, it's hard to find a middle ground between writing about mental illness in an inclusive and encouraging way and addressing the hardships and daily labour people with mental illness face daily. AS IT IS saw that the more you glorified mental illness, the more you indulge in it and find yourself slipping and falling fast.

So his band made it their mission to break this cycle and build a new legacy. In 2018, they released their third studio album, The Great Depression. This album took less of a perspective on asking for help (which was the focal point in a previous album) and more on the receiving end on how to help those who ask. This is a real kick in the ass for other bands and society itself because we hear these artists and fans screaming for help yet nothing seems to be changing. Patty blatantly states "we saw it with Chester Bennington" who was the singer of Linkin Park who tragically took his own life in 2017.

AS IT IS's song, "The Stigma (Boys Don't Cry)," is a perfect example of how society is failing those with mental illness, specifically men. Stigma around mental illness in society makes men seem like failures if they talk about their feelings: "It's better not to say such things out loud." There is this misconception that men should be strong, never let anything get to them, and god forbid…cry: "Don't let them see you fall / Stay strong / Hold on / You've got to keep it together now." Toxic masculinity is rampant in society, which causes an entire half of the population to bottle up their feelings until it's too late.

Another song is "The End.," which the band wanted to keep open for interpretation, but seems to consist of a blatant call for help, which is not properly received on the other end. People may be listening to you, but they aren't hearing what you are saying: "Nobody's listening / Nobody's listening / Straining our lungs to be heard / Nobody's listening / Nobody's listening / Losing our way in these words." This seems like it could be referencing back to the bands who are writing this music like Chester Bennington of Linkin Park. Everyone knew what Bennington was singing about, it was a clear cry out and we understood why… yet, he was unable to get the help he needed.

Fourth wave emo is a considerably smaller scene, however, they were able to touch on subject matter like depression, addiction and other mental illnesses in a much more responsible manner. Songs have less to do with esthetic of cutting yourself and more to do with getting real help like therapy.

The Wonder Years have been discussing mental health issues since their debut album, The Upsides, where lead singer, Dan Campbell, approached anxiety, depression, growing up, touring, and college life. Their next two albums also touched on Campbell's struggles with depression, with songs like "Don't Let Me Cave In" on Suburbia, I've Given You All and Now I'm Nothing, and "The Devil In My Bloodstream" on The Greatest Generation.

In 2015, No Closer to Heaven continued the trend of touching on this deeper content. Campbell pays homage to a friend he lost to suicide, and the struggles that came with continuing to record and tour while dealing with the trauma. No Closer to Heaven is one of the most mature and renowned albums ever produced in the emo and pop punk scene. Albums like this are what pushed other bands beyond the novelty of emo music and started releasing their honest feelings and experiences.

Dan Campbell's song "Cardinals," covers the feeling of regret he felt after ignoring a loved one who needed help and desperately wanting to make up for it: "So if you call be back and let me in / I swear I'll never let you down again / I know the devil you've fighting with / I swear I'll never let you down again." He continues down the rabbit hole of shame, singing about how depression is no easy fix and requires a lot of treatment. Unfortunately, seeking that treatment is an equally tumultuous experience due to the stigma behind it: "Staring at the hole in your chest that's been dug for decades / American promises / Caught between the lies you've been fed / And a war with your bloodstream."

Another band that changed the direction of mental illness in pop punk is Real Friends. Their newest album Composure is another mature step in the right direction, finally avoiding his previous cliches like "i'm a sad boy with boney knees." Lexus Jacobs, a music reviewer from Call The One admires the fact that the lead singer, Dan Lambton, "is not afraid to open up about the dark cloud over him while creating this record." Lambton has previously talked openly about his struggles with bipolar and addiction while on tour. While scrolling through other albums reviews the number one thing mentioned was how refreshing his unapologetic vulnerability was. This was what people want to listen to. Even some journalists who admitted to not loving the idea of emo music, found themselves listening to the album on the daily.

Lyrics in songs like "From the Outside" and "Smiling on the Surface" have tropes on the difficulty keeping yourself together for the sake of those around you. We can assume Dan Lampton is talking about his struggles with Bipolar in most of his songs. Bipolar is most effectively treated with medication, but in "From the Outside" he addressed the uncertainties that come with treatment when you are mentally ill. "From the outside, I seem fine / On the inside I'm still sick / The pill's a temporary fix" shows that even though he is on medication, there will always be an illness and that illness will always challenge the way he is able to navigate through his own mind. This shows the battle of keeping composure (ha, get it) on the surface while dealing with inner turmoil.

When you think your whole world is ending and then that one song comes on — we all have that ONE song — it changes everything. Suddenly, tragedy seems further away, not gone, but away for a while. Suddenly, you feel not so alone, like someone gets you and understands. Suddenly, you feel...saved. When researching for this chapter I went straight to the source: The Defend Pop Punk Group. I simply asked "when has pop punk music been there for you most?" I got a slew of responses but one stuck out to me most:

"I had a pretty shit year recently. I failed all my classes at my uni, my dad had a major stroke, my dog had to be put down, and my ex dumped me. I had so many different artists and albums on repeat. Copacetic by Knuckle Puck and Overexposed by Sleep On It were/are the two I found myself listening to the most. I think this scene has a lot to offer when it comes to getting the shit end of the stick in life. A lot of my favourite bands/albums/songs all share similar qualities. I find myself either feeling less alone and relating more to these artists that I essentially idolize, or being lifted up by their lyrics to remind me to keep my head straight. Not to be sappy, but I'd say this scene is probably a big reason that I'm even typing this right now. I don't think I'd be here without it."

Like, damn. This openness is what this whole book is about. I don't know this person, they don't know me, but this scene allows for people to be genuine and open. This music, these people, it is unlike anything that has ever existed in the music industry. In an era of high stigma, there is a safe place for people to connect and talk about how they feel through a common ground outlet: music.

Now, we don't want to overly criticize the "this band saved my life" mentality that exists in the Defend Pop Punk Group because honestly, it is true to some extent. The scene does great things for people by connecting them with others in similar struggles and offering an expressive outlet for mental illness, which can alleviate pain. However, it is also important to talk about because people in the emo scene tend to sell themselves short when discussing their mental health. Yes, you found support within the bands you listen to, but did they drive you to the doctor today? Did they brush your hair this morning after a week-long episode? Did they remind you to eat today? No, you did that for yourself.

So, is it the band saving you, or are you saving yourself?

This idea of bands saving their fans puts them on a forced

pedestal. Motion City Soundtrack's lead singer, Justin Pierre, jokes in an interview that fans would message him about how much they admire him for being open with his OCD and social anxiety disorder. However, Justin didn't even know he had social anxiety or OCD! He was just "barfing" out lyrics about how he was feeling. It wasn't until years later after going to therapy that he realized he had these things.

Justin appreciates that his music can help his fans, however, he doesn't want to be put in this position of being brave or strong for talking about his mental illness because that wasn't the case. There wasn't thought behind what he was doing so he can't take credit for it. His fans are the strong ones, they are the ones that made him aware of his mental illness. So, when fans message him about saving their life, he wants them to know that the band didn't do anything. They (the fans) were just in the right place, at the right time and heard something that connected with their feelings, but they are the ones that took control themselves.

Patty Walters, again, brings up this unhealthy connection that can happen between bands and mental illness. In an interview for CelebMix, he explains that the reason the bands left the Great Depression album to interpretation is because he wanted the fans to recognize how strong they are even without music intervention. He says "I would love for the people to truly feel, appreciate, and be elevated that they've saved themselves instead of this band." At the end of the album the poet character could have killed himself or not, it is a choice that everyone makes everyday.

Lots of bands in the emo scene offer a lot of support for their fan base. Whether it is raising money for mental health fundraisers, protecting fans in overpowering crowds, answering fan mail, or just writing good music. Many are trying to be open with their own life to show that no one is alone. And while music will always be there for you, in the end, no one is better at saving you than yourself.

Fifth Wave: Emo but with 808s This Time

Recommended Listens:

1. Numb / Encore - JAY-Z, Linkin Park
2. Soundtrack 2 My Life - Kid Cudi
3. Youphoria - Mac Miller
4. XO Tour Llif3 - Lil Uzi Vert
5. Bodybag - LiL Lotus, Cold Hart, Nedarb
6. One Eight Seven - Senses Fail
7. crybaby - Lil Peep
8. The No Seatbelt Song - Brand New
9. ALONE, PART 3 - XXXTENTACION
10. I'm Still - Juice WRLD
11. Misunderstood - Hella Sketchy
12. Betrayed - Lil Xan
13. forget me too - Machine Gun Kelly, Halsey

As the underground popularity of fourth-wave emo passed its peak, a new faction of the genre was gaining steam with an unlikely influence: hip-hop. Hip-hop and rock had seen some convergence from the 1990s to the 2010s, with acts like Rage Against the Machine, Linkin Park, and Kid Cudi, but never in a tangible wave of artists. In the 2010s, this changed. At this point, hip-hop, which dominated mainstream music and the Billboard Hot 100, had pivoted to include vulnerability and weakness as popular song topics, in contrast to its history of braggadocious or resistance-based lyrics. With the embrace of confessional style lyrics by mainstream rappers such as Lil Wayne, Eminem, Kanye West, and Mac Miller, and the fusion of rock-inspired beats and pop hooks by artists like Casper, Yung Lean, and Kid Cudi, the stage for emo rap was set.

During the mid to late 2010s, a wave of new, young rappers, primarily situated on the website SoundCloud, arguably began the fifth wave of emo, known as emo rap. While fourth wave emo is still playing out (having arisen only a few years ago in the early aughts), it is clear that fifth wave emo is a more culturally relevant and visible movement and will likely become the new face of the genre, if it hasn't already. Case in point, emo rap has catapulted in popularity, growing 292% in 2018, according to Spotify's trend expert, Shannon Cook. Some of these artists have achieved or even surpassed the mainstream popularity of third-wave emo artists, with monikers like Lil Peep, Lil Uzi Vert, and Juice WRLD having become household names.

The beats in emo rap songs are laden with guitar licks influenced by (or even directly sampling) second, third, and fourth-wave emo. For example, the track "Bodybag" by LiL Lotus strips the lead guitar line from the Senses Fail song "One Eight Seven," and surrounds it with hip-hop ambiance, replacing the acoustic drums with 808s. Lil Peep's "crybaby" gives a similar treatment to the track, "The No Seatbelt Song," by third-wave emo's Brand New. The amount of "rapping" present in this music is relatively obscure, with artists opting for more melodic deliveries that bounce along to rhythmic, repeating cadences, combining conventions of trap with emo.

The lyrics of emo rap heavily revolve around feelings of anxiety, depression, and relationships. One of the genre's most popular artists, the late Jahseh "XXXTentacion" Onfroy, famously said his album was a "collection of nightmares, thoughts, and real-life situations … and if you are not willing to accept [his] emotion and hear [his] words fully, do not listen." It is a statement that well-defines the emo rap movement — confessional style lyrics that layout self-deprecating thoughts and anxieties to the tune of millions of youth ears. Mental health issues comprise the primary lyrical tropes of the genre, even more so than third and fourth-wave emo.

However, instead of building on the evolving and poignant discourse of fourth-wave emo, fifth wave emo seems to be repeating some of the pitfalls of third-wave emo when it comes to mental health. The fact that most emo rappers take their influence directly from the most popular third-wave emo and hip-hop artists may explain this unfortunate outcome. For example, Juice WRLD had a great affinity for third-wave emo, citing Escape the Fate's album, Dying is Your Latest Fashion as his favourite album, and expressed an interest in collaborating with Buddy Neilsen from Senses Fail. While lamentable, this overlooking of the fourth wave is not entirely surprising, given that the cultural reach of third-wave emo far eclipsed their immediate successors.

Whatever the case, the result is that while fifth-wave emo undoubtedly breaks down stigma regarding the disclosure and acceptance of mental health issues, it also highlights artists, many of whom are the same young age as their listeners, who are not handling the topics very responsibly. A prime example of this recklessness is XXXTentacion's song, "Skin," which contains the lyrics, "Offense or defence, passive or violent / I'll cut my wrists 'til my heartbeat is silent." XXXTentacion then uses this lack of regard for his own life to say that he has nothing to lose in committing violent acts against a man who got in the way of his relationship. In another series of tracks, "ALONE," the rapper postures there is no escape to his depression and inner-turmoil. This sort of content may legitimize critics of the genre who say that the cohort of rappers is creating a culture where depression and suicide are fashionable and incurable, rather than issues that require professional treatment.

One could criticize third-wave emo similarly, but emo rap introduces new problems to its discussions of mental health issues at scale. At the crux of Juice WRLD's song, "I'm Still," is the notion that even though his ex-lover is no longer there for him, pills will always be for him to lean on in hard times, as the singer repeats, "You can't feel, I feel, you can't feel, I feel / Bitch, I still, I still love my pills, Advils." This track highlights a worrying development in emo rap's discourse, which is the notion of using drugs, particularly opioids, as an escape from the heartbreak and mental health issues they have been so forthcoming about. Drug abuse has long been at the forefront of hip-hop lyrics, but emo rap's focus on depression and anxiety may result in the abuse of anti-depression and anxiety drugs rather than cocaine or marijuana. Of course, the use of these drugs also has to do with the proximity of emo rap's audience to the opioid epidemic, rather than opioid-use being a direct symptom of emo rap. Still, the genre is ultimately complicit in the glorification of these substances. The repercussions have already been devastating as several of the genre's most popular rappers, such as Lil Peep, Hella Sketchy, and Juice WRLD, have died early in their careers due to drug overdoses from painkillers like Xanax. Lil Peep was 21, Juice WRLD was 21, and Hella Sketchy was 18.

With its unabashed discourse of mental health, emo rap is uniquely positioned to vaporize the stigma of mental illness amongst its listeners; however, at its current juncture, the prominence of deeply problematic lyrics show the need for growth amongst the genre's flagship artists. Unfortunately, many artists wishing to expand the breadth and angle of their approach to mental health topics will have to do so despite their brand, many of which are synonymous with a cycle of depression and escapism. In the age of social media visibility, adherence to a brand is a 24-hour job. This constant people-pleasing is necessary because successful musicians in 2020 need to create content regularly. What exactly that content is can vary greatly, but it's typically some sort of live video, social media profile, or direct means the artists use to connect with their audience. Consequently, some emo rappers may find that continually playing into their image has altered their psyches permanently. When audiences essentially expect public figures to adhere to their brand image at all times, having an association with partying mental health issues away is plainly problematic, as fans of the band may expect their artists to remain in poor mental health in order to stay authentic. Those rappers who wish to break away from their public persona may struggle to find new attributes to replace their brands' old hallmarks, failing to connect to their audience meaningfully and ultimately risking their livelihood.

Yet, in spite of these potential pitfalls, many of these artists have begun to step up and advance their discourse of mental health issues. One notable example is Lil Xan, who, in the aftermath of Lil Peep and Mac Miller's deaths, has publicly decried opioid use and is attempting to leave behind his own addiction (this, despite his moniker being a direct reference to Xanax). Now, Lil Xan's songs, such as "Betrayed," feature more progressive lyrics like "Xans don't make you / Xans gon' take you," and audiences know him for discouraging opioid use during his performances.

Further, according to Xan himself, he isn't the only emo rapper attempting to move past opioids. In an interview with the Guardian, emo rap producer Nedarb Nagrom said, "after Peep died, a lot of people stopped partying every day. The younger kids don't do stuff as much, because they see all the shit that happened in the last few years." Should this honest discussion of the aftereffects of prescription drug addiction continue, emo rap may be better poised to talk about mental health than any genre before it.

Evolving mental health discourse to the same level of fourth-wave emo at the scale and influence of fifth wave emo would stand to make a massive impact on the lives of many young fans. We hope that these emo rappers will complete the arc of mental health in emo music that originally began in the 1980s. Yet, despite this need for improvement, during the time frame that emo rap has risen into prominence, mental health has become a less taboo subject across all music genres. It could very well be that emo rap has played a pivotal role in bringing mental health discourse in music to where it is today.

PART FOUR: THE AFTER EFFECTS OF THE SCENE

Increasing Rapport for Group Support

Recommended Listens:

1. Adam's Song - blink-182
2. Bro Hymn - Pennywise
3. Check Yes, Juliet - We The Kings
4. Fat Lip - Sum 41
5. Grand Theft Autumn / Where Is Your Boy - Fall Out Boy
6. Bad Reputation - Joan Jett & The Blackhearts
7. Hard Times - Paramore
8. Miles Away - Memphis May Fire, Kellin Quinn
9. Figure Me Out - The Summer Set
10. Dead & Buried - A Day To Remember
11. Go To Hell, For Heaven's Sake - Bring Me The Horizon
12. Identity Disorder - Of Mice & Men
13. Empty Space - The Story So Far
14. Composure - August Burns Red
15. Existence - August Burns Red

In the last section, we ran through the emo movement briefly and considered each movement's relation to mental health. By ending with emo rap, which is still in a nascent stage, we seem to be suggesting that the outcome of emo turned out poorly. It looks like we are suggesting that fifth-wave will culminate in drug addiction and unhealthy coping mechanisms. However, emo rap has not even begun to culminate, and we are just now seeing the rise of a new generation of emos who will likely follow a similar pattern of maturation as third-wave to fourth-wave did.

In contrast, the after-effects of emo do not end in more musical genres. More long-lasting and experienced members of the scene began establishing networks of organizations, support groups, and festivals dedicated to mental health. Support groups within the alternative music/emo scene started to gain traction at festivals like Vans Warped Tour (1995 to 2019), Riot Fest (2005 to present), and So What?! (2008 to present), when people started setting up outreach tents at festivals that provided community support and resources like suicide prevention, abuse support, crisis lines, addiction counselling, and much more. These small booths have since grown into official support websites and international foundations.

Vans Warped Tour came to be in 1995 from a partnership between Kevin Lyman, an event promoter, and Steve Van Doren of Vans. The tour was a melting pot of skate culture and the punk rock music scene, both of which were fresh scenes at the time. Warped was the first tour hosting motocross and BMX sports, and they really went for it. They had bikes jumping ramps over stages and crowds, sometimes the artists performing interacted with the skaters on setups near the stage — like when the frontman of The Aquabats jumped up on a half-pipe, grabbed a skaters board and attempted to do a trick… which resulted in him eating it and the crowd going wild.

Lyman hired artists from a diverse range of genres to perform, intentionally blending and crossing genre boundaries. Although Warped performances consisted primarily of punk and rock, artists like Eminem, Ice T, Black Eyed Peas, Limp Bizkit, Kid Rock, and even Katy Perry "before she was Katy Perry" made appearances, attracting a uniquely broad audience. Those appearances all happened between 1995 and 2000. Warped Tour was always more than punk rock.
To combat the "rockstar ego," Lyman would change the schedule every day and not give it to anyone until the morning, thereby removing the idea of a tour headliner. He and his team were dedicated tour managers and promised the artists travelling with

them that there would be worldwide tours if everything went as planned. And there were. Warped Tour was the first tour to travel worldwide, hosting Europian, Hawaiian, Belgium, Japanese, Germany, Barcelona, UK, and Australian tours. The tour in Australia was nearly inconceivable. Lyman convinced bands that, at the time, were selling millions of records — blink-182, Pennywise, The Vandals, 311, Reel Big Fish — to camp in one big dirt field, in tents, where they brushed their teeth and washed their hair with bottled water. The worldwide tours were a massive success.

Warped Tour started with two stages. But the side stages' success was wildly unexpected. Eventually — and it changed all the time, sometimes more than once during one summer's tour — there would be 5, 6, 7 stages. There was a "Smart Punk Stage," an "Ernie Ball Stage" where We The Kings first played at Warped. There was a "Kevin Says Stage," where bands would go up to Kevin and tell him they wanted to play. He would say, "if you show up, you can play Warped Tour." So they would show up to production and demand that "Kevin said if we showed up today, we could play." Lisa Brownlee, Warped manager and one of the first female tour and production managers in the industry, would say, "that's not a thing." The whole ordeal amalgamated into this crazy, big, sponsored stage. Many bands blew up at these side stages, attracting larger than expected crowds and getting a significant kickstart to their career. They would go from smaller side stages to larger ones, and eventually to the main stages. Among these bands who got their first big breaks on Warped was Sum 41, Fall Out Boy, and Maroon 5.

There was a Nightly BBQ for the performers and crew members, which often included fans and tour attendees. Every band and crew member gathered around a giant BBQ, with an unlimited supply of beer and food, creating an atmosphere to decompress. The people that attended these BBQs believed they were a spot where people connected the most. As Matty Mullins from

Memphis May Fire puts it, "it was an opportunity just to get to know people. Instead of being like 'hey, I'm in this band,' it was more like, 'how are you doing, bro?'" Everyone had opportunities to befriend people they probably wouldn't have known or met otherwise. Every year, Lyman would offer for bands to come on Warped Tour, except that they would have to transport the BBQ and cook for the feast. If they did a good job, Kevin put them on a stage. So they got a chance to play by paying their dues.

> "What you're doing for that band is massive. They're so grateful, and they're so stoked to play, and you're so stoked to see them have this rad experience," is how Ryan McLain, the Ernie Ball Experiential Director, puts it. Steve Van Doren sees the BBQ as "a big way to get the family together."

Additionally, Warped had a strong female leadership behind the scenes. These women knew better than anyone how male-dominated the rock world is. While experiencing this first-hand, if there was a female band to book on a label, they booked them without any doubt. Save Ferris, Joan Jett, Hayley Williams & Paramore, Juliet Simms and PVRIS were all promoted by Warped. They worked hard to create a comfortable and accessible environment for women to connect.

Offstage during Warped Tour were side hustles that, over time, turned flea market. The way to survive while on tour was to hone a skill or provide products and services that you could sell. There were guys selling water bottles, people who would pull a wagon around backstage filled with iced coffees to sell to everyone, crew members who sold set schedules for a toonie. One guy sold disposable cameras, killed it, came back a few years in a row, and got hired to be a part of the tour. There were jewellers, dunk tanks, and lots of t-shirt tables, some of which weren't even band merch. These side hustles grew and turned into a real flea market that set up at every stop. This punk-rock atmosphere created a community like no other.

The Entertainment Institute came to life throughout Warped, and Lyman believed that the initiative would have "Warped Tour [become] the largest classroom in America." Starting as a way for artists to better connect to their fans, those artists would work to run education programs backstage. Artists held classes on everything from drumming, guitar lessons, bass lessons, even harmonica lessons. Jess Bowen from The Summer Set offered a drumming class that she aimed for female participants because it's uncommon to see female drummers. Lisa Johnson, legendary rock photographer, hosted a 60-minute one-on-one photography class, taking students right into the pit for firsthand experience. The Education Institute provided opportunities for fans to learn from people who love their jobs. Artists would talk about songwriting, social media, building brands, how to get into the music business, or how they got their start. Matt Halpern from Periphery remembers fondly how some parents would approach them to say, "I haven't seen my kid happy in so long — because somebody told them they can do this." This exchange of knowledge and appreciation also inspired artists to give motivational speeches in the institute, which naturally bled into their live performances.

The crew went so far to create a community, that when they started noticing some parents were scared of them and would wait outside the venue for their kids to leave, they created "Reverse Daycare." The motto was for kids to check their parents in, while they go watch and have a good time. The space was air conditioned, had bean bags, water, tables, lounge chairs, and tv screens. It resulted in more parents feeling comfortable with their kids going to the show.

Warped Tour was fan-friendly, catering with low ticket costs and easily accessible attractions. It was an event that brought like-minded people to one central location and often felt like a world fit for outcasts. It was a place where bands first started seeing people get tattoos of their lyrics, and where fans and artists alike got to exchange thank yous. It was a welcoming affair, run by strongly motivated (mostly female) crew members, who held strong inclusion values. Warped was the type of event and community that, when friends, brothers, and loved ones passed away, a song would be dedicated and sung to them by the entire band and audience, creating an uplifting environment for artists and kids alike. Pennywise would play their song "Bro Hymn" and bring the person who's lost a loved one onto the stage, letting them sing the song. Jason Thirsk remembers those times vividly, when "the emotion that person had while singing that song would bring tears to your eyes." Whether it was coming together to mourn or facing a nasty storm, everyone worked together and helped one another — it was like a family. Everybody was there to lift you up no matter what. That's what families do. To make a show happen, they grew together through challenges and did whatever it took to get those artists in front of fans (safely, of course).

Universally, attendees, crew members, and artists remember Vans Warped Tour as a monumental game-changer in an abundance of ways. For many, there was nothing like it. As Joe Sib, a Warped crew member from sideonedummy records, and Steve Van Doren point out in interviews, all Kevin Lyman wanted to do was give people opportunities; he could provide 400 to 500 bands a year a chance to feel like a rockstar. People who attended look back and see Warped as a "turning point that they got to start being their true individual selves, out in the world," as Jen Kellogg, co-founder of the Education Institute and tour accountant, would put it. Warped — and the people behind it — promoted inclusion and breaking the rules while still being respectful. Tour crew members Steph Mirsky, Dave Atkinson, and Kate Truscott believe it was a place for people to be themselves and inspired them to take that into the world because you don't need Warped Tour to be yourself. You could be the jock, the misfit, the skater or punk rocker; you could have neon hair, be gay or straight, it didn't matter. It was a place where "kids who didn't feel normal, were able to feel comfortable." Many hard-working individuals put their best efforts into making that true of Warped Tour year after year.

So, if Warped Tour left a legacy of inclusion, self-reflection, education and awareness, loving what you're doing, respecting others, and much more, you must be asking yourself what they inspired and left behind. There must be proof, right? Well, yeah. There sure is. Activism was a major component of the tour and allowed for non-profit organizations to advocate their causes. These groups advocated various issues surrounding everything from cancer awareness and fundraising to anti-harassment and sexual assault awareness. These include (but are not limited to):

- Invisible Children, Inc. (2004 to present)
- Shirts for a Cure (2002 to present); Keep a Breast Foundation (2000 to present); "i love boobies!" donation bracelets; Girlz Garage (tent during warped tour, and a side-tour featuring female bands, including Canadian act Lillix).
- Music Saves Lives (2006 to present)
- EarthEcho International, Inc. (2000 to present) ; Rock the Earth (2002 to present)
- PETA(1980 to present)
- Hollywood Heart(1995 to present)
- Our Music, My Body (2016 to present) who partnered with Riot Fest! to co-write the first anti-harassment policy for the concert
- MusiCares (1993 to present)
- A Voice for the Innocent (2014 to present) who, in 2016, teamed up with Warped Tour to address the issue of sex crimes in the music scene.
- To Write Love On Her Arms ; Hope For The Day ; Heart Support (which we'll dive into soon).

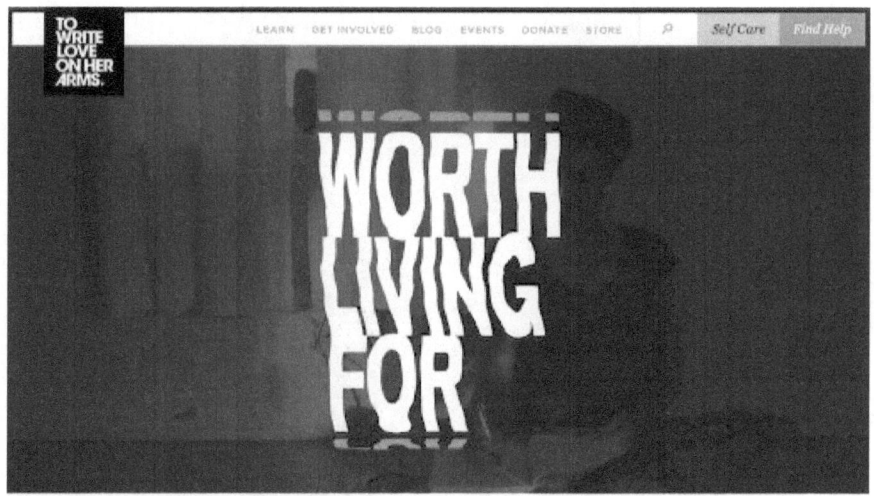

Warped Tour was the genesis of outreach tents in festival culture. It paved the way to a culture that created and inspired countless other festivals, concert tours, support groups, non-profit organizations, and more. Everyone from artists to event promoters started to aim for growth within the scene by self-reflecting, acknowledging wrong-doings, and putting proactive precautions into play.

One festival that followed Warped was the Self-Help Fest, put on by Jeremy McKinnon from A Day To Remember (ADTR). The goal behind it was to create a safe haven community to listen to music and to focus on one crucial thing: self-help. As McKinnon explained, following a conversation with his girlfriend, "most people who come [to our shows] respond like it's more than just a concert to them. It's like the music is genuinely helping them. Thus, we titled our festival Self Help, because at the end of the day that's what music's all about." Self Help Fest launched its first installment in 2014 in San Bernardino, California, alongside acts such as Bring Me The Horizon, Of Mice & Men, The Story So Far, Memphis May Fire, Atilla, The Word Alive and many more. They later followed it up with a northeast date in Philadelphia that same year, and have continued hosting the festival every year since.

In an ALT Press interview, McKinnon tells us his favourite thing

Late One Night, Jake Luhrs Sat Outside The Chicago House Of Blues

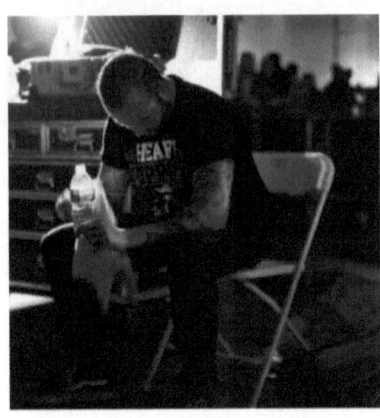

Stories of addiction, depression, self-harm, heartache, war, fear, and hopelessness echoed in his mind. Every night, a fan would share a different story.

Although Jake was the well-recognized frontman of August Burns Red, he was at a loss for how to help. He wasn't a mental health specialist and he screamed into a mic for a living. *Not exactly the picture of expertise his fans needed.*

Deep in thought and prayer, all Jake knew was that something had to change.

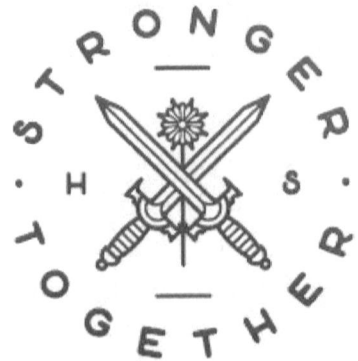

DIVINE INSPIRATION STRUCK

And That's When He Got His Answer

- Build a place where people can come exactly as they are and explore healing
- Provide relevant resources to an increasingly digital generation
- Teach them to give back and help others grow **stronger together**

about the festival is "the reaction from fans and bands alike. The crowd has been over the top into all the bands every year so far. Really pushing the performances to another level. Then on the bands' side, it's awesome just to see people having a good time and feeling like they're being taken care of. That doesn't happen in our genre at the moment." These thoughts bring to light an important observation that the founders and members of outreach programs make — it's a starting point for self-reflection in the scene to be better every day, every show, every meet and greet. ADTR built Self-Help Fest from the ground up with a positive message inspiring it and having the bands' and fans' best interests at heart.

Hope For The Day (HFTD), one of the outreach programs listed above, started in 2011, in Chicago, by Jonathan Boucher. He was a booking agent who, after losing 10 friends and family members to suicide, decided to start this non-profit. He grew up just north of Chicago and got involved in the music industry at age 13 by putting on punk metal shows while creating community spaces where people felt they could belong. "HFTD is a non-profit movement empowering the conversation on proactive suicide prevention and mental health education." Through outreach, education, and action, they aim to "equip people with the right tools to be proactive in their communities." They believe and preach that "together, we can break the silence around mental health." They spread the message that "it's ok not to be ok" globally, and have representation in 50 states, 26 countries, and 17 languages. They offer options to get involved by providing educational resources and social platforms to share stories and connections, including downloadable and shareable resources, and selling merchandise to purchase that funds are donated. They also have an option to become an "Agent of Impact;" an individual who is committed to shattering the silence of stigma in their community.

HFTD partnered with Dark Matter Coffee to create a coffee shop, the first of its kind, "Sip of Hope." 100% of the proceeds support proactive suicide prevention and mental health education. They also created a matching coffee blend called "Sip of Hope," with printed mental health resources on the bag, and sell them in their shops, online, and in select stores. "Sip of Hope is the perfect space for breaking the silence around suicide and raising the visibility of mental health resources in our community." The coffee shop staff is non-clinical, as the shop is not a drop center, nor do they treat & diagnose. However, they are trained in a non-clinical crisis interventional program, "Mental Health First Aid," that is offered by the American Foundation for Suicide Prevention. This way, they can still create a safe atmosphere to relax, rewind, and make connections you'll remember for a lifetime. Sometimes, their therapy dog, Tesla, visits the shop to comfort customers in need of a little furry-friend pickup. Like the non-profit itself, the coffee shop aims to break stigmas and silence surrounding mental health and is powered by the love of music and safety within its scenes borders.

To Write Love On Her Arms (TWLOHA) was another program listed above. In 2006, Jamie Tworkowski wrote a poetic letter telling the story of a friend - Renee Yohe - who was struggling with addiction, depression, self-injury, and suicidal thoughts. After convincing her to go into rehab, they denied her because she was too high risk, so Jamie housed her and provided a make-shift rehab until a program willing to help admitted Renee. Jamie sold t-shirts to pay for her rehab treatment, starting in the scene he knew and loved - the music scene, especially rock, punk and emo. He posted his story on MySpace and sold shirts out of a booth at every show he could attend, rapidly accruing wide recognition in the music world and being supported by popular bands like Paramore, Switchfoot, and Anberlin.

Quickly realizing he had stumbled into a conversation that he couldn't ignore, he asked himself how he could help those who were struggling. In 2007, TWLOHA became an official non-profit organization. "TWLOHA is a non-profit movement dedicated to presenting hope and finding help for people struggling with depression, addiction, self-injury, and suicide. TWLOHA exists to encourage, inform, inspire, and invest directly into treatment and recovery." The organization has shared the message of hope and help with: 210,000+ messages responded to over 100 countries around the world. They have travelled 3.8+ million miles to meet people in their communities. 1,100+ blog posts shared and launched a podcast (with 300+ episodes) - to let others know that they aren't alone. Since 2018, their "Find Help Tool" has seen 56,000 program searches, and for every four searches, someone will take the next step to sit with a counsellor or call a crisis hotline. The "Self Care" tool provides countless tips and connections to find hope and get help. $2.4+ Million donated to treatment and recovery, including granting funding to 105 unique organizations and counselling programs.

Last but not least, a third program that has, and still is, making waves in the emo scene - HeartSupport. A community created by Jake Luhrs of August Burns Red, where people discover the strength to overcome suicidal thoughts, depression, addiction, and other adversity. Started in 2013 as just five good buddies with the heart to help, they created it as a place for kids to share and rant their experiences and struggles without judgement. They weren't counsellors, and it wasn't therapy, it was just outreach community support intended to connect kids to websites and resources that might help them, and counsellors in their area when necessary. After years of fans thanking him for saving their lives with his music, hurting for them, and wondering what he could do to provide help more substantially and professionally, Luhrs found the solution he sought.

"By creating relevant recovery and support for an online generation, HeartSupport has been recognized as a leader in the industry winning non-profit of the year at the APMAs in 2016 and named as one of the Top 100 Socially Innovative Non-Profits in the World in 2017. We believe no one should struggle alone and aim to create a world where music fans find the encouragement, support, and products they need to take their next steps without fear, shame, or judgment," their website reads.

HeartSupport has grown into a full-fledged organization, partnered with doctors and psychologists to provide resources to those seeking help. Their website (and Discord, Twitch, Instagram, Twitter and Facebook) provides access to resources that are researched and developed by a team of certified mental health professionals. Dr. Gretchen Wolfe, Dave King, Nate Hilpert, John Williford, Dr. Michelle Saari, Dr. Justin Halcomb, Dan, Meagan Prins are among these team members. Additionally, Taylor Palmby, their media coordinator, is a certified Crisis Line

Responder; Ben Sledge, an ex-military who is working on an advanced diploma in Crisis Response, Trauma Care, and Suicide Prevention from Light University that focuses on combat stress, PTSD, and moral injury and "work with veterans for a new initiative with HeartSupport." Casey Keys (CaseyScreamsBack) is a faithful father and husband, and a supporter for self-care and mental wellness, who is a content manager of HeartSupport, including running a Twitch stream discussing mental health awareness related topics near-daily.

There are various resources and tools available on their sites. These include depression and anxiety email support signup and downloadable workbook, a digital support wall based on the original Support Wall created at the 2018 Vans Warped Tour where you can talk to peers. There's a text support line (text the word "heartsupport" to 512-647-2871), or join a livestream and chat through Twitch, where CaseyScreamsBack & DanMakesHisMark host people like Matty Mullins from Memphis May Fire to share their experiences with anxiety, depression, mental illness. They offer even more than that, providing tools for loneliness & relationships, addiction & self-harm, and sexual abuse on their website.

A few other notable mentions that have been vital to the music scene: The Jason Foundation (1997-present); SoundMind (2018-present); RecoveryFest (there are a couple versions of this); the Tour Health Research Initiative (Started in 2020); and the Send Me A Friend Foundation (2017-present).

"Mental health, anti-harassment, environmental awareness and sobriety now have a place at festivals, providing fans with ways to get involved and give back to the world around them while still enjoying the music." Every individual who participates in this music scene and loves it the way most fans do, work to improve it. These artists, event agents, and fans mentioned, among important others, work tirelessly to improve the dialogue between music and mental health.

Everyone is Emo Now

Recommended Listens:

1. High Hopes - Panic! At The Disco
2. P.S. I Hope You're Happy - The Chainsmokers, blink-182
3. Irresistible - Fall Out Boy, Demi Lovato
4. I Think I'm OKAY - Machine Gun Kelly, YUNGBLUD, Travis Barker
5. 1-800-273-8255 - Logic, Alessia Cara, Khalid
6. I Love Me (Emo Version) - Demi Lovato, Travis Barker
7. OK Not To Be OK - Demi Lovato, Marshmello
8. ocean eyes - Billie Eilish
9. everything i wanted - Billie Eilish
10. Nightmare - Halsey
11. Gasoline - Halsey
12. Girlfriend (Dr. Luke Mix) - Avril Lavigne, Lil Mama, Dr. Luke

After decades of emo musicians getting chastised ironically for their overemotional take on music, mental health discourse moved into mainstream genres in a palpable way. Not only did the emo scene outlive the criticism, but it fortified into one of the most influential and popular music genres to date (2020). Fashion trends may have moved from coon tail streaks to egirl curtains, but the genre and alternative style continue to stay relevant. Let us be clear; emo is alive and well.

Third-wave emo band, Panic! At The Disco, skyrocketed to the #1 spot on Billboard's Top Rock Songs with their 2018 song "High Hopes" for a record-breaking 65 non-consecutive weeks.

The weeks were non-consecutive because their other hit song, "Hey Look Ma, I Made It," reached the #1 spot as well for 11 weeks! Panic! At The Disco is an emo band that stayed true to their foundations while evolving to attract a wider audience, which many others started to follow. blink-182 collaborated with The Chain Smokers, Fall Out Boy has a song with Demi Lavato, and blink-182 drummer Travis Barker has produced for Machine Gun Kelly, YUNGBLUD, and a legion of young hip-hop artists. The emo sound has diverged into multiple streams of music and influenced others to push the boundaries of lyrical content in their own music.

Not only do we see traditionally emo artists broadening their sound for mainstream media, but we are also seeing mainstream artists bringing in emo sounding elements, and perhaps not so coincidentally, speaking about mental health on a broader scale. Popular artists like Logic, Halsey, and Demi Lavato have all taken a mental health activist approach with a lot of their music.

Logic had an emotional performance at the 2017 MTV VMA's singing his Billboard Top 100 song, "1-800-273-8255." After the awards show, there was a 50% spike in the volume of calls to the National Suicide Prevention Lifeline within hours. This spike was mainly because the name of the song just so happens to be the hotline phone number. Logic's massive platform helped spread the awareness of the available resources for mental health crises that would maybe not be known to everyone. He also took into consideration who would perform the song with him at the award show. Instead of glamorizing the song with back up dancers, crazy lights, and elaborate costumes, he brought up 50 suicide survivors to participate in the conversation. He made it accessible and casual with hooks like "Who can relate? Woo!"

This song is sung from the perspective of a depressed and desperate individual calling the helpline and speaking with an operator. The first chorus is the initial confession to the operator, "I don't wanna be alive, I don't wanna be alive / I just wanna die today, I just wanna die." The second chorus is the operator trying to soothe the caller, "I want you to be alive, I want you to be alive / You don't gotta die today, you don't gotta die." This change in dialogue is a breath of fresh air because, sometimes, a distressed individual just needs to hear that someone, anyone, cares about them. It doesn't always have to be coming from someone in your immediate cohort. Even a stranger's compliment or support can go a long way for someone going through a crisis. The last chorus is the caller coming to terms and accepting their help, as Logic sings, "I finally wanna be alive, I finally wanna be alive / I don't wanna die today, I don't wanna die." Many people may feel anxious about getting help, but approaching the topic lyrically in a catchy rap song makes the process seem easy and less intimidating.

The song also features other elements that can accompany mental illnesses, including stigma ("And my life don't matter, I know it, I know it / I know I'm hurt deep down and can't show it"), loneliness ("I never had a home, ain't nobody callin' my phone / Where you been? Where you at? What's on your mind? / They say every life's precious but nobody cares about mine"), and despair ("I've been praying for somebody to save me / no one's heroic.") Logic explained that he wrote the song for those who lack emotional support from their parents and parental figures who are supposed to be the ones they can turn to. Instead, you can turn to daddy Logic — he's got you.

One artist who candidly opens up about their struggles with mental illness is Demi Lavato. Demi has been transparent through social media and interviews about her trouble with alcohol, cocaine, self-harm, bipolar disorder, and eating disorders. She also released a documentary entitled "Stay Strong," where Demi shares her story about the process of learning she was bipolar. While her original diagnosis was a hard pill to swallow, she has continued to be honest about her experiences and understands that discussing it through her music may push others to seek help.

A lot of her lyrical content is about empowerment and support for those who are suffering, including songs, "Skyscraper," "Yes I Am," and most recently (released during Suicide Prevention Awareness Month), "OK not to be OK." However, she also has songs from a more personal space involving her struggles with addiction and trauma, including "Warrior" and "Sober."

"Sober" is a melancholic melody which she wrote after relapsing for the first time after six years of sobriety. She discusses the symptoms she felt while trying to get sober, "Call me when it's over cause I'm dying inside / Wake me when the shakes are gone / And the cold sweats disappear / Call me when it's over / And myself has reappeared." In interviews, Demi has explained the difficulty of getting sober the first time. She had gone on various campaigns promoting sobriety despite the fact she was continuously relapsing — a truth she admitted to in "Sober:"

> "Momma, I'm so sorry, I'm not sober anymore
> And daddy please forgive me for the drink spilled on the floor
> To the ones who never left me
> We've been down this road before
> I'm so sorry, I'm not sober, anymore."

Her song "Warrior" makes references to possible childhood trauma: "There's a part of me I can't get back / A little girl grew up too fast / All it took was once, I'll never be the same." Many fans speculate that it could be about her father sexually abusing her because of the blaming nature of the lyrics: "I need to take back the light inside you stole / You're a criminal / And you steal like you're a pro." Whatever her reason for the song, many fans take solace in the lyrics. Everybody has or wants to overcome some form of hardship in their lives, whether it is self-harm, addiction, abuse, or some form of disadvantage. The song is a reminder that no matter what life throws at you, you are strong and capable of handling it: "Now I'm a warrior / Now I've got thicker skin / I'm a warrior / Stronger than I've ever been."
Eventually, she does forgive herself and accepts that she is only

one person and can't be perfect; she can only be a human being, and humans are flawed. Marketers, managers, and media outlets tend to censor artists like Demi Lavato, who start on platforms like The Disney Channel when sharing about their personal lives. For instance, Bella Thorne had come forward about being terrified of photos of her kissing her boyfriend leaking online. This kind of control forced Demi to hide her addictions and mental illness from the public for years. However, she now has the capability and freedom to share her experiences with people around the world.

The media-proclaimed "sad boy" aesthetic became popular around 2013 when SoundCloud rapper Yung Lean rose to prominence. This new wave has since taken over everything: social media, including fashion, influencers, and artists of all kinds. Emo music influenced many modern-day artists with their musical style and lyrical content.

Nevermind Hannah Montana, forget Justin Bieber, the newest teen pop sensation is Billie Eilish. This neon green, chain-covered pop princess has swept the music industry, winning numerous awards and recently winning all four main categories at the 62nd Grammys at just 18 years old. These achievements were not won solely by Billie but instead with the help of her brother Finneas O'Connell. Finneas has written and produced every single one of Billie's songs that she has released. Both Billie and Finneas have mentioned in interviews that they both take a lot of influence from bands like Green Day, My Chemical Romance and Fall Out Boy. All of which Finneas grew up listening and exposed to Billie.

Finneas originally wrote her hit single, "ocean eyes," for his band, The Slightlys, who played numerous festivals, including the ultimate emo summer camp you will remember from earlier: The Vans Warped Tour. Now, we wouldn't classify Finneas' band as an emo band, but being a dude in a pop-rock act surrounded by the Warped emo culture, we can see where he picked up some influence for Billie's music. His producer for The Slightlys, Eric Palmquist, has also worked with numerous emo bands including

Thrice, I the Mighty, and Never Shout Never. Given the content of Billie's music, it is likely that Finneas' exposure to emo subculture played a role in shaping the sound of her music. It is all to say that Finneas has nailed the formula between alternative and pop sounding songs that cater to the divergent and disaffected teens that make up most of Billies' audience. This is the same audience that identified with emo during the peak of its popularity in the early 2000s. Her signature sound and lethargic esthetic formed a new class of emo fan that has become more attractive in the mainstream media than ever before.

Billie Eilish is a perfect example of how emo culture manifested itself into the mainstream music we hear on the radio today. As Gen Z's most influential mental health advocate, Billie talks genuinely and openly about her struggles with mental illnesses. While doing an interview with The Gayle King Grammy Special, she was brought to tears when discussing her experience with suicidal thoughts. She admits that she did not know if she would make it to 17 years old and encourages her fans to reach out for help before taking that extra step.

Further, during an interview with Rolling Stone, Billie explained that her music is about darker subjects like suicide and depression because she wants her fans to know that they are not the only ones out there "feeling like shit." While her reasoning can seem juvenile (which she is), it helps spark conversation in the music scene just like third-wave emo did. She has songs about anxiety, drug addiction, and losing friends to suicide. Considering she is still a teenager, Billie is making an impressive impact in the music industry. Her progression is eerily similar to Avril Lavigne's career, and no surprise, Billie is a huge fan.

Her song, "everything i wanted," is a chilling trap beat where she paints a picture of herself feeling so insignificant that if she were to kill herself, no one would care. In it, Billie sings, "So I stepped off the Golden / Nobody cried." In interviews, Billie explains that she wrote this song about a bad dream and how her brother can always help her when she is feeling vulnerable. However, the analogy behind the lyrics could be taken as the perspective of celebrities calling for help and the world either ignoring them or patronizing them for their feelings: "I tried to scream / But my head was underwater / They called me weak / Like I'm not somebody's daughter." We can reference this back to Patty Walters discussion about celebrities outright screaming for help and society ignoring them, like Chester Bennington.

Many people seem to continue to discredit Billie's feelings and mental health. Because she is so young, all the Karens and Richards out there believe she hasn't had enough life experience to know what depression is, or what anxiety is. This kind of toxic outlook from the older generations is dangerous for younger generations. According to the non-profit youth suicide awareness and prevention program, The Jason Foundation, suicide is the second leading cause of death for youth ages 12 to 18. Children and teenagers need to know that their feelings are valid. They shouldn't be degraded for struggling with mental illness by those who should be guiding them and helping them through it.

We still stand with this young queen for continuing to talk about these challenging subjects, even in the face of adversity. Celebrities who have these conversations on their large platforms can do so much good for the world. She may be young, but she is changing the conversation once again, just like many emos before her.

Halsey is another mainstream artist who has taken some major inspiration from the emo scene. Pre-fame, Halsey would film herself singing covers on her YouTube channel, including songs from blink-182 and Sleeping With Sirens. Nowadays, she has collaborated with mainstream scene figures, like emo rapper Juice WRLD, blink-182 drummer Travis Barker, and emo rock band Thirty Seconds to Mars.

Rest assured, Hasley was in the mid-2000s emo trenches just like the rest of us. The influence steeps deep after years of listening to pop-punk artists like All Time Low, The Story So Far, and Panic! At The Disco. Halsey has tweeted about religiously attending Warped Tours throughout her life, and in 2019, they invited her to play for their 25th-anniversary concert. What a win, Queen.

Her song "Nightmare" features the classic emo sound with distorted guitar, nu-metal-esque drum beats and a wicked deep threat scream. The music video even featured the punk fairy godmother herself, Debbie Harry, the lead singer of Blondie.

We are here supposed to be talking about her songs involving mental health topics, but we just had to stop for a second because this song is THE BOMB. Now back to our regularly scheduled programming.

Halsey is known for participating in advocacy for suicide prevention, sexual assault survivors, racial injustice, and women's rights. She boldly uses her platform for social causes and has always been genuine about her mental illness struggles. For example, Halsey opened up about bipolar disorder in a series of YouTube videos for Mental Health Awareness Month. She got the participating licensed therapist, Dr. Snehi Kapur, to explain to her fans what bipolar is and provide resources for those struggling with it. She admits she previously attempted suicide when she was 17 and describes how she ended up in a psychiatric hospital for just over two weeks. We are all vulnerable. Even celebrities who seem perfect have their flaws.

In her song, "Gasoline," Halsey opens up about her bipolar disorder and some of the side effects that tend to appear. Her lyrics, "are you insane like me? / Been in pain like me?" and "Do you call yourself a fucking hurricane like me?" might not be the most clinical terms, that's for sure, but she is referencing her manic episodes. Halsey relates that she experiences spending binges during her episodes. She alludes to this symptom, singing: "Bought a hundred dollar bottle of champagne like me? / Just to pour that motherfucker down the drain like me." She talked about her manic overspending in interviews before, explaining that she stayed in a castle and took a red wine bath when she was on her first tour at 19 years old. The above lyric directly correlates with her mental breakdown during that tour. She sings about this episode in her full-length debut Badlands.

Her album titles and content, like that of Badlands, mimics her Bipolar disorder episodes. Badlands and Hopeless Fountain Kingdom are both depressive periods; both are worlds different from one another. Manic follows her high-energy and sporadically fleeting moments of making whatever she "felt like making; [because] there was no reason [she] couldn't make it."

There are also more thematic elements to her song that are less to the point. Her life has the potential to spiral like the champagne she is pouring down the drain. Her lyric, "would you use your water bill to dry a stain like me?" is Halsey asking if people are willing to put up with her insanity, even when it leaves a mark behind. In interviews, she explains that sometimes she feels like an "inconvenient woman" because of her mental illness, but owns it anyway, and wants to let others know you can still live a full and happy life.

Halsey has taken over the pop world as one of the most insightful lyricists at just 25 years old. She has sold out arenas, scored a number one hit on Billboard's Top 100, and has dropped three studio records. Halsey is exceptionally impressive, to say the least, and continues to grow as an artist every day. Hopefully, she continues this lyrical quality and her unconditional activism for those at a disadvantage in society.

While there is still a tremendous amount of criticism and negativity around musicians that are politically active and discuss mental illness, the mainstream music world has made steps towards a better future for artists. During a time of intense stigma, emo musicians broke the norm of lyrical content to make music about mental health and emotions. In return, it rippled out into mainstream society and changed how we think about mental illness today. We are now seeing mainstream artists take this courage and bring it into their respective scenes to continue the conversation. The emo scene's goal continues to be about defending those who feel alone, marginalized, or emotionally distressed. They will not go quietly into the night. Well, they will, but they will bring a pair of headphones and jam out to emo tunes walking off into the starcrossed and moonlit horizon.

Pretty brave, in my opinion.

The Crown Jewel: Musical Therapy

Recommended Listens:

1. Good Riddance (Time of Your Life) - Green Day
2. The River of Dreams - Billy Joel
3. My Girl - The Temptations
4. Let It Be - The Beatles
5. Hallelujah - Jeff Buckley
6. Fix You - Coldplay
7. The Climb - Miley Cyrus
8. Change the World - Eric Clapton
9. Blue Suede Shoes - Elvis Presley
10. All Star - Smash Mouth

Music therapy emerged as a clinical science since the early 1900s. However, music therapy's first practitioners may have predated David and King Saul I, who used music in a variety of ways to relieve grief and suffering.

Notwithstanding ambiguous history, music itself is comforting, relational, and at times challenging and confronting. These aspects of music are inherently therapeutic and transcend clinical and colloquial contexts.

Nowadays, music therapy utilizes musical performance, listening, and composition to promote physical and emotional healing and wellness. Clinical music therapy is only delivered and curated by a certified music therapist with a relevant graduate degree and accreditation from a regional college of musical therapy. This accreditation requirement upholds the professional and scientific integrity of the discipline.

The jury is no longer out on music therapy's efficacy; it works tremendously for treatment, and ongoing management of several debilitating conditions. However, academics still debate why and how music therapy benefits patients; the exact biological mechanisms acted upon by music therapy are generally unknown. This ambiguity has cast doubt on the therapy's scientific validity and true clinical efficacy. Nevertheless, consistent patient outcomes implicate music therapy as a cornerstone treatment for a variety of physical and mental conditions.

Examples of clinical significance

- May improve memory deficits and cognitive function in dementia and alzheimer's disease
- May reduce subjective pain ratings of chemotherapy in cancer patients
- Can treat PTSD symptomology in children and adults
- May improve sleep duration and sleep quality in insomniacs
- May improve speech dysfunction in patients with apraxia

Music therapy often crosses diverse genre boundaries. For example, music therapy may take the form of singing in a choir, improvising rhythms in a drum circle, or simply humming a pleasant tune with a music therapist. These activities are intended to allow patients and practitioners to explore social, cultural, and psychological issues that underpin a person's conditions.

Music therapy: our scientific understandings

Music therapy is among the most powerful of alternative therapies for neurorehabilitation after brain injury. While some brain injury sufferers may find sound of any kind intolerable, it is often reported that particular pieces of music are soothing to these patients. Regardless of a brain-injury patient's tolerance for sound, music therapy is considered a front-line treatment option to improve brain function deficits while promoting physical healing of damaged tissues and substrates.

Specific musical therapy treatments have shown to be efficacious for treating localized dysfunction of specific brain regions. For example, engaging with rhythm (toe tapping, hand clapping, dancing to music, etc.) has been shown to have beneficial effects on somatosensation and motor coordination in TBI sufferers with cerebellar injury and parietal brain-bleeds. Emotional expression, considered a coordinated function between subcortical and cortical substrates, may be improved through practicing musical improvisation. Damage to lateral-temporal and lateral-frontal areas associated with speech production and comprehension has been shown to improve with singing and vocal breath work.

> "Neuroscience reports successful outcomes with specially engineered music therapy programs. Reports of music making a difference abound in science and classical literature. In Bible days, musicians were sent ahead of Warriors to maintain morale and to set the climate of victory for battle. Recently there has been much emphasis given to the Mozart effect. In some studies, music has been emphasized as being able to even enhance mathematical ability."
>
> *- Amy Price, Ph.D*

Broad collections of research endorse music therapy as an effective pain-management strategy. Postoperative patients receiving musical therapy in combination with treatment as usual had significantly lower opioid requirements for managing post-operative pain.

> "In three studies evaluating opioid requirements 2 hours after surgery, subjects exposed to music required 1.0 mg (18.4%) less morphine (95% CI: -2.0 to -0.2) than unexposed subjects.

Additionally, in five studies assessing analgesic requirements 24 hours post surgery, the music group required 5.7 mg (15.4%) less morphine than the unexposed group (95% CI: -8.8 to -2.6)."

- *Journal of Practical Pain Management, Volume 12, Issue 5*

Music therapy's analgesic properties have also been observed in cancer patients undergoing chemotherapy; decreasing subjective pain ratings by as much as 70% in some patients.

Music therapists must use careful discretion when prescribing a musical treatment plan. Musical protocols must be designed intentionally, so as to alleviate specific forms of pain; it is not a "one size fits all" approach.

Part of the therapist's job is to empower patients to identify music that speaks to them on a personal and spiritual level; teaching them how to engage with music in such a way that arouses multiple sensations simultaneously. This engagement involves coordinated activity from multiple brain areas, and is intended to create a meaningful diversion from the perception of physical pain. Techniques such as singing, playing instruments, rhythm work, improvisation, listening to music, and composition may be used individually or concurrently to achieve specific treatment goals.

Anxiety reduction is often a foundational starting-point for pain cessation. Music therapy has shown to reduce anxiety in patients with mental health diagnosis' and detrimental physical conditions like metastatic cancer. This reduction of pain associated with anxiety is shown to originate predominantly from quality of life improvements. Understandably, relief from health-related anxiety is bound to associate with a wide variance of positive health outcomes — however, blunted perception of physical pain is considered an unexpected by-product of music therapy by physicians, therapists, and patients.

Music, whether an active or passive experience, impacts sensory perception. Music serves as a diversion, sanctuary, and shield for people experiencing many forms of pain. A key determinant of music therapy's efficacy is a musical intervention that resonates with a patient's specific needs. This includes careful consideration of musical selections, activities, and rapport building between patients and therapists. Music therapy is eloquent in it's cost effectiveness and efficacy to improve a broad range of health outcomes. The harmful side effects of music therapy are few, and generally under examined by medical researchers.

Music Therapy and Mental Health

Music is a universal human experience. Music's healing potential has been recognized by most fields of medicine, employing nearly every musical genre and delivery form. This practice has evolved from a traditional social-science approach; one that focuses on health and well-being, toward a neuroscientific approach that examines specific musical elements and their effects on sensorimotor, linguistic, and cognitive functions. The handful of evidence-based music therapy studies on psychiatric conditions have shown promising results.

Several meta-analyses have evaluated short to long-term effects of music therapy on schizophrenia patients compared against their usual treatments. Generally, there was a positive effect on their symptomatology and prognosis'. Music therapy improved 'negative' symptoms (characterised by dampened affect, disposition and behaviour), quality of life, and social functioning when compared against control groups. More specifically, regularly scheduled music listenings may reduce auditory hallucinations, while rhythmic based music theory has well documented efficacy in reducing the severity of prodromal states - the precipice that often precludes a psychotic break.

Positive results in music therapy interventions for schizophrenia are most often associated with increased functional connectivity in the dorsal anterior insula, posterior insula, and frontal cortical areas. While these improvements can be observed through functional magnetic resonance imaging (fMRI) after only one month of music therapy, the improvements do not typically sustain for longer than six months.

Music therapy is often combined with medications, psychotherapy, and other therapies to increase the efficacy of treatment programs for schizophrenia, anxiety, depression, and other mental health conditions.

CONCLUSION

Well folks, there it is. We've traversed the murky seas of emo music to try and clear up the water a bit.

We hope to have given some evidence that supports a few things:

First, on the whole, mental health historically has not had a centre stage role in mainstream music until the rise of emo music.

Second, emo music itself evolved in terms of its mental health conversations. The first two waves began explicitly addressing mental health more than punk music had ever before. The third wave exploded into the mainstream, making its relation to mental health varied between artists; but overall, it concerned bringing the conversation to table. All three of the first waves also had messy relationships with mental health, often expressing emotions surrounding mental health but not addressing how to get better. Further, as the moral panics exaggerated beyond reality, there were cases of artists offering suspicious and ambiguous songs that may be interpreted (or misinterpreted) as toxic for young minds. However, this criticism could be leveled against any form of musician that misuses their platform. Additionally, emo artists were developing, confused, and emotionally distressed teenagers learning to navigate the world. It's not surprising that, when such intense emotions come openly from a youngster, they sound extreme to an adult who might be unfamiliar with mental health and its expression.

We then wanted to show that fourth wave emo took note of their complicated situation in the media and amongst their fans. This recognition led bands to try and accurately depict mental health-related topics without glorifying or stigmatizing mental illness. More importantly, it reminded its listeners that taking action about mental health is important — and it became more relatable by dropping the rockstar attitude and sex-symbol look. Artists began recognizing their ineptitude to actually save lives and began putting onus on the listeners and fans to actively pursue real mental health and treatment in a clinical setting. They became supporters of the fans' choices to save themselves, rather than saviors coming to rescue their audience from mental health struggles.

Part four looked at the impact of emo music on the dialogue of mental health in society. We ran through the festival community, which provided resources of all sorts to fans who wanted to engage more with mental health. This discussion led into a walkthrough of a fraction of the support groups that blossomed out from emo culture and talked a bit about their influence and success. Next, we returned to popular music to see how emo artists have become lasting figures in popular culture. We checked back in with pop music to see it has taken on an obsession about mental health again and explicitly cites emo music as an influence. Finally, we looked at music therapy in clinical settings to see how music is beginning to settle neatly into the clinical world.

Now, if we are successful, readers have managed to get a sense of the emo movement and have begun to think about our suggestion — that emo was a contributing factor to the present prevalence of mental health conversations across all forms of media. With any luck, readers will now wish to investigate individual artists, topics, events, and questions that we have discussed and they will have reference material to return to. Historical, musical, and literary analysis about emo music is dreadfully lacking in the academic world, so there is plenty of opportunity for students in the humanities or literary departments to explore heretofore unexplored territory.

That territory is filled with questionable fashion, cringeworthy photos, awkward teenagers, angst, sadness, and anger. Yet it is also filled with compassion, love, empathy, beauty, and personal strength. It also yields a treasure mine of links to major contemporary conversations. It's also cool. You want to be cool, right?

www.ingramcontent.com/pod-product-compliance
Lightning Source LLC
Chambersburg PA
CBHW030117170426
43198CB00009B/650